PREGNANCY PRIMER

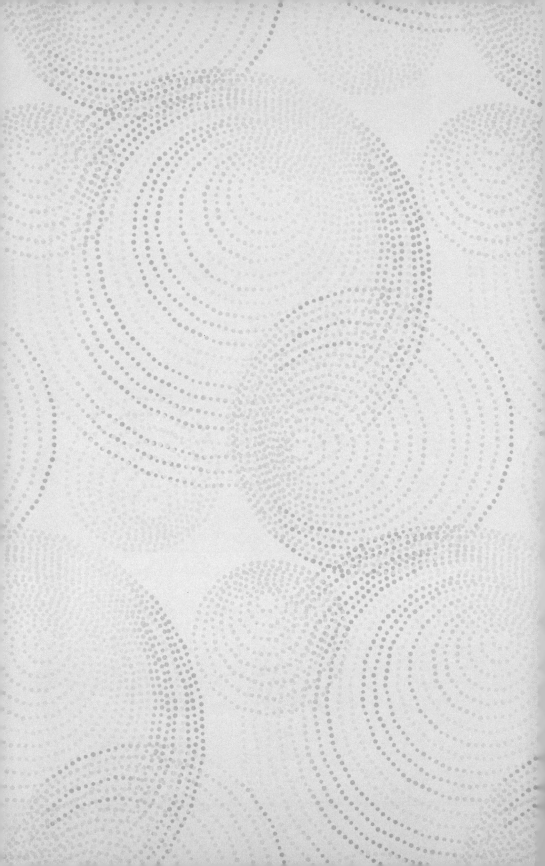

the
PREGNANCY PRIMER

THE EXPECTANT MOTHER'S GUIDE TO ALL 9 MONTHS

MELANIE J. PELLOWSKI

Author of *My Dearest Bridesmaid* and *My Dearest Sister*

Skyhorse Publishing

Skyhorse Publishing books may be purchased in bulk at special discounts for sales promotion, corporate gifts, fund-raising, or educational purposes. Special editions can also be created to specifications. For details, contact the Special Sales Department, Skyhorse Publishing, 307 West 36th Street, 11th Floor, New York, NY 10018 or info@skyhorsepublishing.com.

Skyhorse® and Skyhorse Publishing® are registered trademarks of Skyhorse Publishing, Inc.®, a Delaware corporation.

Visit our website at www.skyhorsepublishing.com.

10 9 8 7 6 5 4 3 2 1

Library of Congress Cataloging-in-Publication Data is available on file.

Cover design by Laura Klynstra and Daniel Brount
Cover illustrations by Melanie J. Pellowski and gettyimages

Print ISBN: 978-1-5107-4585-8
Ebook ISBN: 978-1-5107-4586-5

Printed in China

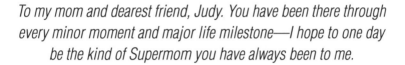

To my mom and dearest friend, Judy. You have been there through every minor moment and major life milestone—I hope to one day be the kind of Supermom you have always been to me.

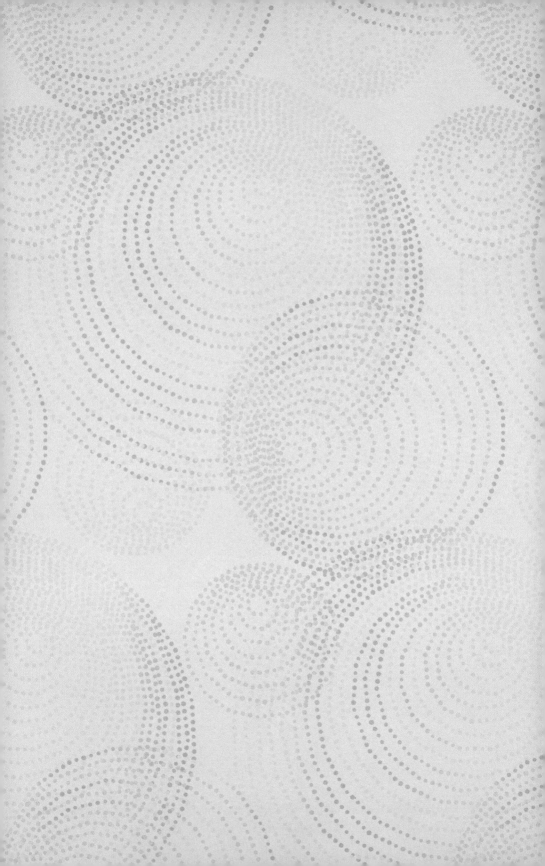

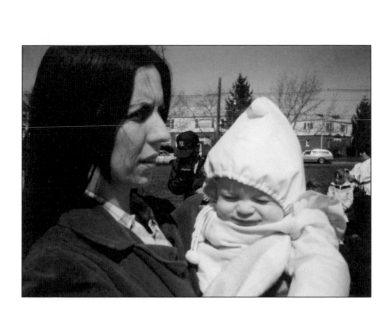

"When my first child was born, we didn't have all of the technology afforded today. I still don't know if I would want to know the sex of my child before it was born. Every time my obstetrician would tell me it looked like I was having a boy, and with my third child, I remember in the delivery room him saying, "Well, we have a cheerleader here!" I was excited, of course, at first to have a healthy baby, but really excited because I had a baby girl!"
—Judy

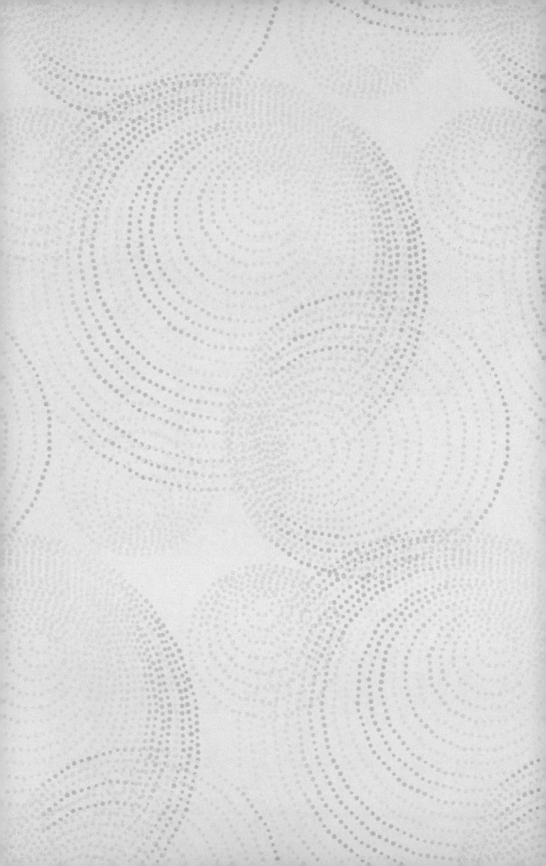

Table of Contents

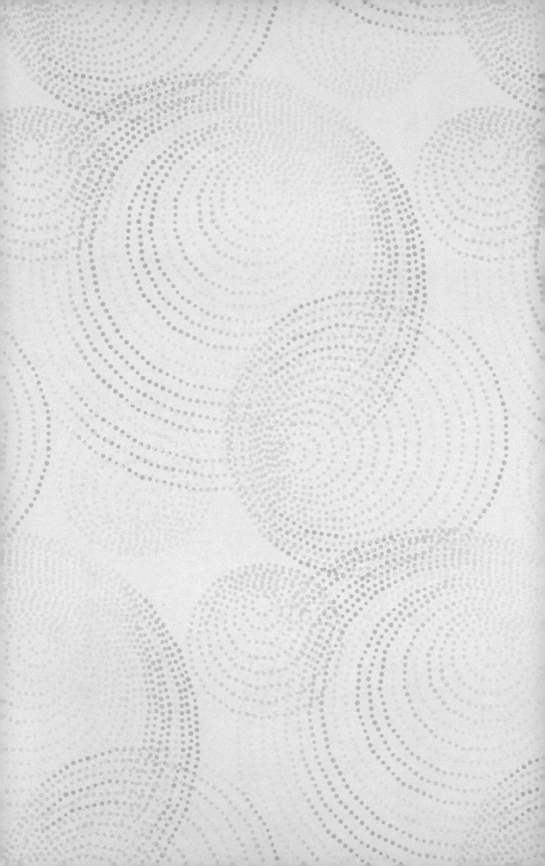

A Note for Mommies-to-Be

We mommies-to-be sure are a special bunch. We come in all shapes, sizes, and ages. We have nothing to worry about and everything to be concerned about. Is that why we're queasy? Call it nerves, anxiety, or biology—our bodies are built to handle it, and our minds are, well, filled with ideas, hopes, and dreams!

Our personalities are peculiar, unique, and let's just say it, totally awesome. But our pasts are our own and we might have different ideas about how to approach this weirdly beautiful, somehow manageable, definitely challenging, hardly perfect, but absolutely heartwarming and rewarding pregnancy journey. We can all agree that it's obviously a blessing, but everything else might be up for discussion. So, how do we get through it without losing our minds, our sex appeal, and ourselves?

Fret not, future moms—we all have our own tale of how we became beautiful women, and we'll write our own stories as we become mothers too. We aren't the same, but our futures have something in common: we're all about to give birth to the cutest baby of all time!

BORN TO BE A MOM

Some of us were born to be mothers. We carried a reproductive spark in our genes before we even understood how babies are made. As little girls, we cared for our baby dolls as if every imaginary breath hung in the balance of how we held a plastic bottle or pushed a pretend stroller. We adorably rocked our little doll dumplings, dressed them up, changed their diapers, and treated them as the real deal.

It's telling how we took care of those pretend babies by feeding them fake food from our shopping carts or rock-solid cookies baked fresh from our Easy-Bake Ovens. We were the most legit mothers-in-training and probably should have earned a badge, ribbon, or Girl Scout patch signifying our accomplishments. We had an innate aptitude for parenting as adorable big sister helpers who cared for our younger siblings in the cutest of all ways.

We have longed for the day when we could carry our own, when we too could fulfill our destinies as devoted caregivers. Truly, everything else we have done in life was merely a prelude in the story of who we were fated to become. We can hardly contain our excitement when we see a baby's tiny feet—we can't help but smell their stinky toes and like it! We are psyched to become parents and hardly feel complete before we give birth to a smaller version of ourselves. We are the women who already know, deep within us, that becoming a mother will be our greatest achievement and most valuable role.

REBORN AS A MOM

Some of us women are anxious to be mothers. For whatever reason, we might have always wanted to have children one day, but suddenly the reality of that "one day" dream crept up on us, as time typically does. We look at pictures of ourselves and don't understand the lines that have formed near our eyes. What the heck is that, anyway? Stupid crow's feet—must be a shadow. The same time-space conspiracy that shrunk our jeans in the dryer.

Maybe the giving birth part seems like a harsh technicality of something special. It's not that we timid ladies aren't ready to mother, it's that in our minds we will never be ready, not until the birds and bees fly in and buzz the words, "Hey girlfriend, you have always been ready." Still, it might feel like a sting, not quite the soft transition and life milestone we once imagined in a few fleeting thoughts. We'd get there, one day, and that day is now here. Eek!

Some of us might be surprised to suddenly harbor motherly charm we didn't realize we had, but the mom gene runs in all of our veins. We might be a little nervous, but we worrying types holding onto our pre-pregnant bodies are going to be great moms too. Our sense of adventure must be passed down to the next generation of giggly girlfriends, and we'll be the ones setting the curfews.

RECRUITED FROM ABOVE

Maybe we didn't always dream of mothering. Maybe we thought that being the world's greatest aunt was enough. Perhaps becoming a mother is a mixture of emotions. Sure, it's exciting and beautiful, but also the most terrifying job any woman will ever take. It's more of an internship, really, and our babies have no say in hiring us. They are stuck with us, placed with us by a divine recruiter.

These babies have no idea how lucky they are, do they? What a bunch of little dough balls; we can't help but cherish them. One day, they'll learn the concept of appreciation. They'll remember everything we did for them, and likely the *one* thing we *didn't* do for them. How did our own moms do it? They sure were amazing. No matter what, we are bound to discover this to be the most rewarding, fulfilling, special, and inexplicably purposeful thing any woman will accomplish.

A MOST REWARDING ROLE

Becoming a mother is a mixed bag. It's going to be hard. It's going to be brilliant. At times, it's going to be wretched (but never wicked—save that for the evil stepmothers). It's bound to be exhausting most of the time, and painful many times. It's also going to be lovely, hilarious, magical, momentous, and enchanting. Whether a woman always carried that mommy idea in the back of her brain or even if she never thought she'd be the one to reproduce, every type of woman has the potential to be the best kind of mom. Congratulations, first-time mom, let your pregnancy journey begin and your new adventure continue to be cherished for years to come.

Pregnancy Journal

When I first found out I was pregnant, I:

_____

_____

_____

_____

_____

I am most excited about:

_____

_____

_____

_____

_____

I am most nervous about:

_____

_____

_____

_____

_____

I have questions about:

_____

_____

_____

_____

As a new mom, I hope to:

_____

_____

_____

_____

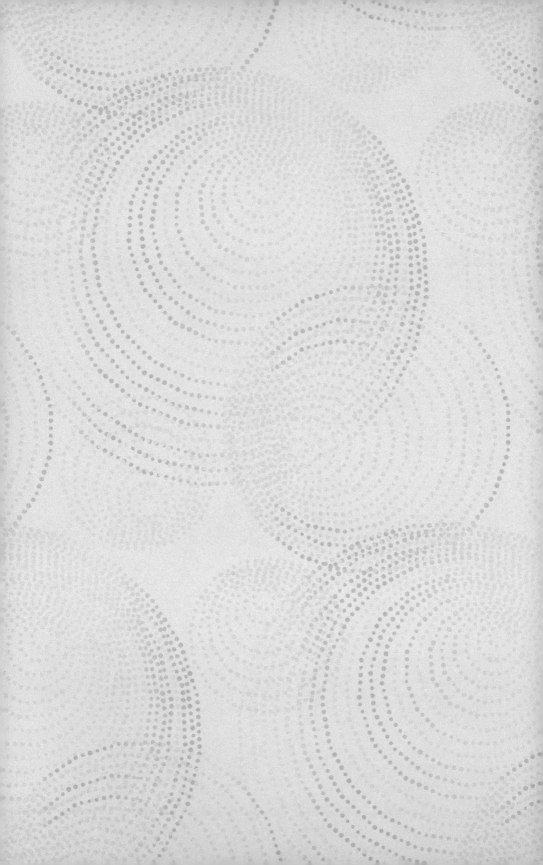

Chapter 1

BECOMING SUPERMOM

There may not be an instruction manual for becoming adults, but there is a lot of information out there to guide us on becoming new moms. Motherhood is basically an extension of all things confusing and we definitely have experience in being confused as grown women! Let us rejoice in the comfort of good company.

THE LEADING ROLE

When most of us were little, we imagined that every adult had all the answers. We dreamt of one day becoming old enough to learn the answers ourselves, but the biggest truth we discovered is that clarity is often a ruse. We Dorothys *have* paid attention to the man behind the curtain, and the reality is that we're all confused about something or other. We put on a confident face and give our best performance, as if we were cast in a play on humanity and are stumbling around without knowing our lines. Whoever is up there watching is certainly getting a good show. "Those women," the audience laughs. "They really try."

We will try—every day for the rest of our lives—to set an example for our children and be the best moms out there. We aren't always going to be the best, though. We are human, after all, and we haven't seen the entire script! Soon, we will have many roles to play, and chances are we'll be winging it most of the time. This is improvisation at its best, baby. Luckily for us modern moms, we have a lot of great resources to help us learn. Time to go to Mom School!

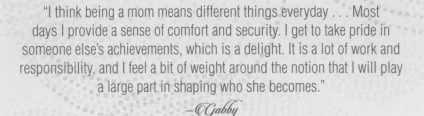

> "I think being a mom means different things everyday . . . Most days I provide a sense of comfort and security. I get to take pride in someone else's achievements, which is a delight. It is a lot of work and responsibility, and I feel a bit of weight around the notion that I will play a large part in shaping who she becomes."
>
> *—Gabby*

NEW MOMS UNITE!

Just as the times have changed and the expectations for moms have evolved, the mothering guide books have entertained new advice and concerns through the decades. Despite the convenience of information being at our fingertips, it's always good practice to double check any medical tips and questions with your own doctor. Triple check these suggestions with your own gut instinct. Seek advice, but don't blindly take anybody else's word for what you should or shouldn't do during your pregnancy. For Pete's sake, please don't just type your symptoms into an Internet browser search! Trust yourself. Ask your mom, your aunt, your grandmother, your girlfriends, your doctors. Take comfort in the fact that a little more than four million babies are born in the United States each year alone! That means you are not alone, sweet mommy-to-be.

> "Being a mom is the closest I'll ever come to feeling like a superhero, and hearing my kids say, 'I love you Mommy,' makes the sleep deprivation, weight gain, and mastitis completely worth it."
>
> *—Anastasia*

SUITING UP

These nine months are more like ten months of training and settling in to becoming your best self—a superheroine, even. Go ahead, take a look in the mirror. The beauty staring back at you is about to get serious, purposeful powers. Perhaps that pregnancy glow is a reflection of your soul fulfilling its destiny! Don't be overwhelmed—be ready. You're on your way to becoming *Supermom*! This is your origin story, whether you decide to wear a maternity mom cape or not. That little nugget nesting inside of you is your life coach, your love, and your creation. First-time mom, you are a blessing, a beauty, and a human being full of life. Be still the worries of your big heart and growing belly. A perfect little human is ready to be your gift to the world!

A BEAUTIFUL BOND

The bonds formed between a mother and her baby start long before hearing that first cry in the delivery room, and they are bound to last a lifetime. You are about to endure the kicks, the cravings, and all that comes with carrying a beautiful little load in your kangaroo pouch up front. Women literally are the vessels that safely transport, develop, and carry the future of mankind and womankind. No pressure though, right? Actually, there's probably some pressure (both literal and figurative), but not to worry: strong women are built to handle it.

There's the beauty of being pregnant and the attractive beast a woman becomes when it's time to deliver. A new mom has a lot more going on within her beyond the baby in her belly. Pregnancy is a wonderful foreshadowing that proves the strength and stamina stitched into the framework of every woman's story.

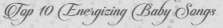

A STRONG START

Pregnancy might not be a cake walk, but it is going to be a journey toward an incredible, unforgettable beginning (and the refrigerator). The understandable fear you feel along this journey will often be quieted by a soft whisper of the truth: the fact that you know that you will be a great mom. No matter what, you just will.

The first time you take a look at your baby's tiny little fingers and toes may generate feelings we don't currently have words for, a moment filled with emotions we cannot describe in written text. There is nothing but our own confusing sensibility that is somehow crystal clear. This precious gift in a blanket is bound to warm our hearts in an instant and those feelings will last forever. The communication and connection you already feel with the baby you carry is mystifying. How do we explain it? It's just, well, super!

"Even with a full life, friends, career, family . . . It's all kind of still about you. When you're a mom, it's the first time the switch becomes not about you and about them. You learn selflessness and it's all worth it."

—*Jackie*

STAGES OF SUPERMOM TRAINING

For now, your superhero development takes place in three stages. The first, second, and third trimesters. It's like having three acts in your own play and you are the star! And even though you have the leading role, you're *encouraged* to gain weight! How great is that? Each stage, or trimester, lasts about thirteen weeks.

FIRST TRIMESTER

Your first superhero trimester begins in week 1 and goes through week 12 of your pregnancy. With your new powers, you may experience the powerful urge to release your bladder—a lot. You may tire easily, not only from all of those trips to the bathroom, but from everything. Caffeine and sugar will likely only make your lethargy worse. It's okay, your body is essentially getting used to the idea of being tired all the time for the rest of your life. Do not be discouraged by this. Be empowered! By week 5 of your pregnancy, your baby has grown from being only a few cells to now being a cute little embryo! He or she is on their way to becoming the president. You can just feel it.

"The most challenging aspect of being pregnant was the nausea during the first trimester and the fatigue. I ate a lot of carbs and took a lot of naps in the beginning. Also, ice cream fixes everything."

– Caitlin

MORNING SICKNESS

Morning sickness is like a diner with rotating doors that serves breakfast all day; it may greet you at sunrise and stick with you through the afternoon and evening. Not every woman experiences morning sickness, but those who do may feel like they are at war with their appetite. There's no real cure or antidote to feeling like you're about to puke, only the sheer will to survive and, well, some ideas to help outsmart your body into feeling better. Staying hydrated and drinking water consistently helps. Avoiding food that has a potent smell is a good bet. *Grease* will always be a good movie but maybe not a good move for your body. Try nibbling on a bunch of meals all day long rather than attempting to keep down one big plate of food. Love up that chicken broth and become a plain Jane for a while. Think of it like a fabulous detox!

SOUNDS LIKE LOVE

Are you thinking about your pregnancy soundtrack yet? Contemplating making a mix tape? In week 10, you may experience your first ultrasound and learn the due date. You also might be able to hear your baby's heartbeat for the very first time. Be still our own hearts! It sounds like love! All of those nauseous feelings melt away as science rocks our minds. Your little one's organs are developing and he or she is on their way to becoming a verifiable little human.

"Hearing the heartbeat for the first time was exciting and surreal! You've been waiting for that moment, but there's this small piece of you that doubts this baby is really happening. Then you hear that rapid beating and you're happy and so relieved."

–Gabby

SECOND TRIMESTER

The second trimester begins in week 13 and lasts through Week 26. There's some exciting stuff happening in this middle round! You may feel the baby move for the first time around Week 16. Plus . . . the placenta is here! The placenta provides the baby with oxygen, nutrients, and waste disposal.

SNAP A SOUNDIE

Will you discover the sex of your baby before he or she is born? Should it be a surprise? We now not only have the capability of sharing every image we'd like with our online followers; we can get a three-dimensional look at the little one all curled up inside of us. Talk about a roller-coaster snapshot! Air traffic controllers have nothing on our ultrasound operator.

IT'S A · · · SURPRISE!

Now that you're off in the clouds thinking about personal touches to put on the nursery, it's a good time to talk with your boss about maternity leave and plans you have as a new mom. Like, bye! I'm never coming back to work. Or, bye! I'll be back soon. No matter what work choice you make, it will be the right one.

THIRD TRIMESTER

The third trimester is the home stretch of your pregnancy. Shout it from the mountain tops! You are going to be an incredible mom! Actually, don't shout too much. Your little one's hearing is developing and they might be able to hear and recognize your voice. Think about your tone and what you say throughout the day. Though the noise will be muffled, your baby will find familiarity in the sound and tone of you or your partner's voice. It's likely you'll be feeling your baby move around a lot too. How cute! Do you have a boxer or soccer player on your hands? Should you get a trophy made to put in the nursery? That's up to you. By the time it's time to give birth, it may feel like it took forever or it might feel like your pregnancy flew by. Either way, try to enjoy each moment and celebrate the finish line with one big push.

"To me, there's nothing greater in this life than being a mom. You can have a career which is fulfilling, but if you are fortunate to have children you have a lifetime of happiness in watching your children grow and experience their lives through your eyes."

—Judy

Pregnancy Journal

I am grateful that my mom:

_____

_____

_____

_____

I admire moms that:

_____

_____

_____

_____

I hope my baby is:

_____

_____

_____

_____

I am happy that:

_____

_____

_____

_____

_____

While pregnant, I hope to:

_____

_____

_____

_____

_____

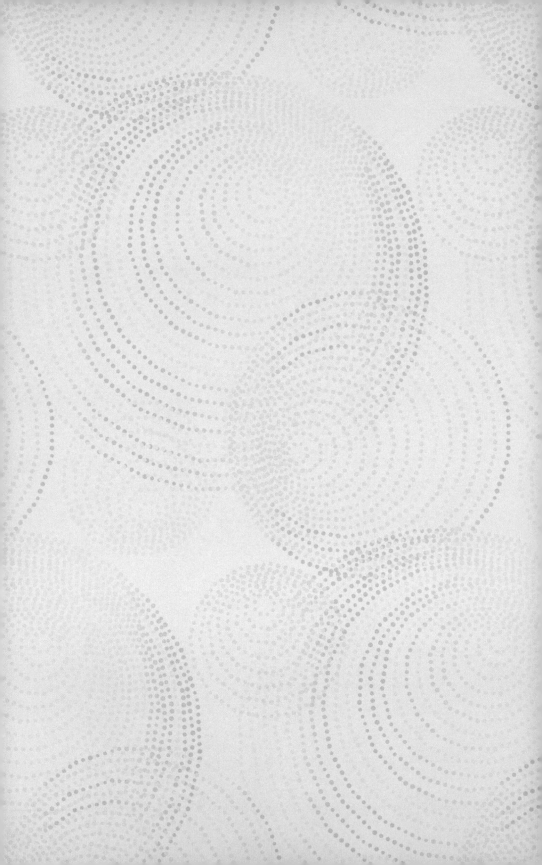

Chapter 2

PRENATAL SPARKLE

This pregnant walk you have stumbled on is your path toward an even more brilliant life, one that is forever intertwined and enhanced by a life you produced through love. Everything is only going to get better, brighter, and . . . well . . . bigger. Transforming into a heightened version of yourself doesn't mean you're going to be perfect. Far from it, actually. It means that you're going to find purpose in being imperfect. You're going to make it work, Mama! You have a long road ahead, but be inspired! Your training begins now, and your life coach couldn't be closer to home.

THE DREAM TEAM

Talk about motivational training. This baby is the perfect excuse to kick-start a healthier lifestyle! Now is the time to reflect and recognize exactly what you are putting into your body and why. Chances are, if it isn't good for you, it isn't good for your baby. What's good for your little one is likely good for you too!

GROWING PERKS

As your belly grows, your knack for walking in a straight line might be derailed and your previously graceful style might experience some bumps in equilibrium. You're not clumsy though—you're elegantly awkward in an impressive way.

Time to put on some big girl pants! As you develop your extremely fatigued superhuman strength as a new mommy-to-be, your body may endure some changes. For example—and this is exciting—your breasts have the potential to quadruple in size! You might also notice that the skin along the midline of your tummy is becoming darker. This is called linea negra, and it's like a rite-of-passage for a pregnant woman. You're the cool new mom with the belly tattoo!

"I felt like a princess, legit. You can do no wrong during a first pregnancy. You could probably get away with murder and everyone would just look around and say, 'well, she's pregnant and probably exhausted! Get that girl some ice cream and a couch!' Yes, seriously."

—Christy

SCRATCHING THE SURFACE

This is all new and you are just beginning to scratch the surface of becoming a great mom. Speaking of that, some pregnant women experience itching all over. It might just be their body and mind adjusting to the concept of gaining super strength. Want something else to celebrate? You can scratch those menstrual cramps off the calendar for the next year or so, and they might not even come back. Nobody ever liked them anyway! Your new powers can also stop the growth of painful endometriosis.

HEIGHTENED SENSIBILITY

Pregnant women tend to have a nose for details and their heightened sense of smell tends to impact what they crave and want to avoid. It's typical for some pregnant women to be grossed out by meat, eggs, and seafood. Wouldn't you know it, these selections are all more likely to carry harmful foodborne illnesses, and Mama doesn't need that drama! It's best to steer clear of stuff like unpasteurized dairy products, raw eggs, undercooked meats, and fish high in mercury.

BITTER BABY

We don't have to be pregnant to be bitter in general, but we're bigger people now. Pregnant women might be turned off by bitter-tasting foods due to their heightened sensibility, and research suggests these aversions could be an evolutionary trait. Toxic fruits and plants have a bitter taste, and some pregnant moms can't bear the smell of alcohol. It's like we have an innate superpower telling us to avoid eating what's bad for us. The good stuff though? We want all of it.

> "I was extremely lucky to feel really well throughout my pregnancy. I'll never forget, however, about spraining my ankle at seven months. The books aren't lying about your center of gravity shifting and being really off-balance!"
>
> —*Gabby*

EAT UP, BABY

Your baby needs sustenance to grow. Eat frequently and graze often. Snacking all day is a good way to satisfy your appetite while keeping it at bay. Your little one needs help growing, and it's your job to facilitate that growth by providing the little sucker with nutrients. Relax into the idea that gaining twenty-five to thirty pounds of baby weight is recommended. Try not to get too comfortable, though, because excessive weight gain could lead to gestational diabetes. Aim for an extra three hundred calories a day, but don't lose your mind counting. You have enough to worry about!

SUBSTITUTE MOM

Try to find healthier substitutions for your favorite cheat meals, and keep in mind that food additives and sugar substitutes should really be avoided. You should always rinse off fruits and vegetables prior to cooking and eating them. A good balanced mix of lean proteins, calcium, whole grains, fruits and vegetables, and healthy fats is a decent start to getting into your healthy mom bod. Eating foods that are high in minerals like iron, calcium, magnesium, folic acid, and zinc will be a good combination for you and your baby to sync up your powers too.

PRENATAL VITAMINS

Prenatal vitamins are no excuse to ignore eating healthy altogether; rather, they are an extension of your heroic transformation. It's like a nutritional booster seat! So, what does a prenatal vitamin typically contain and why?

Folic Acid is important because it reduces the risk of neural tube defects like Spina Bifida. Iodine controls metabolism, along with Vitamins A, B(1), B(2), B(3), and B(6). (Are we new moms or grandmothers playing Bingo? Both options sound fun.) Calcium plays a big part because it strengthens your teeth and the baby's teeth, too, while Vitamin D does its job by coaching your baby's bones and teeth to be strong and fierce. Meanwhile, Vitamin C helps your body absorb the iron it needs so badly. Iron is seriously important because it prevents anemia and assists in the baby's blood development. Vitamin B(12) is good for the blood, too, and copper can also help prevent anemia while aiding in bone formation. Not to be forgotten, zinc helps balance fluids and aids in nerve and muscle function.

WHAT'S UP, DOC?

Doctor's offices can sometimes feel cold, but don't let that stop you from getting comfortable. You are going to get to know one another very well these next few months, during fifteen or so appointments. Expect to be prodded and probed, but don't feel like you're on an alien spaceship. Instead, settle into the fact that you are a human treasure and bring a loved one for support. You'll likely see your doctor once per month during weeks 4–28, then twice per month until week 36, and weekly from then on until the baby is born.

When you have questions, write them down here and bring them with you. That will help you remember what you'd like to talk about, and keep in mind, there are

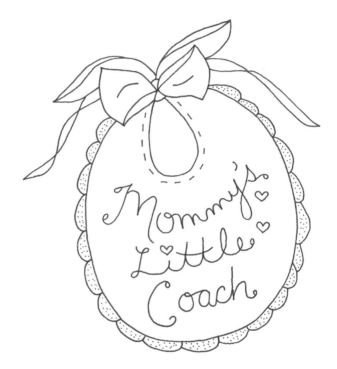

no dumb questions, and it's always better to ask and be reassured about whatever it is that is making you feel anxious. It's not easy becoming a superhero, and doctors are there to help as you learn how to flex your new mom muscles.

Mommy's Notes for Doctor

How have you been feeling? Are you concerned or curious about anything? Keep track of any questions you might have for your doctor by writing them down here.

MOM FLEXING

You might feel some aches and pains along the way, so it's always best to check with your doctor about which over-the-counter medications are safe to use. You should also talk with your doctor about skin and beauty products you typically use to find out what makes the most sense for you and your baby moving forward. You've already got that pregnancy glow, girl, so don't worry if you need to make a few alterations to your beauty regime.

DON'T WORRY, BABY

Yikes. Did you throw back a few beers one weekend before learning you were pregnant? Were you toasting a friend or getting happy at happy hour as adults typically do? Don't worry, baby, you aren't the world's worst mother before you even knew you were going to be a mom. There's no evidence to show that drinking alcohol in early pregnancy can harm the tiny little cells that are barely even an embryo yet.

DON'T DRINK IT, MAMA

Do concern yourself, however, with cutting out booze for the rest of your Supermom training once you know that you are pregnant. Beer bellies are no place for babies and no amount of alcohol is 100 percent safe to consume during pregnancy.

CLEAR THE AIR

There's always going to be a story of a carefree mom who smoked when she was pregnant and the baby turned out fine. Think about all of those lottery winners that keep giving us false hopes of becoming overnight millionaires, though. They're all a bunch of pipe dreams. Smoking is bad for the baby and can lead to many complications in your pregnancy. Be safe, don't smoke. Nicotine is a Supermom's kryptonite!

CLEAN IT UP!

It's a good idea for pregnant moms to be aware of odd odors they are breathing in on a daily basis. If you have the energy to clean the house, be sure to open the windows or ventilate powerful fumes. Wear rubber gloves when handling cleaning supplies or strong products. Think about bringing in some household plants. They add oxygen to the air and suck up other pollutants, not to mention make your place a little cozier and give you practice in keeping a living creature alive. (It won't help you with figuring out how to change a diaper, though.)

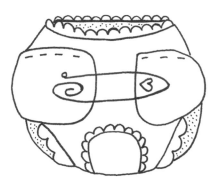

CAFFEINE

Keep in mind that sharing is caring and you share everything you consume with your baby. You don't necessarily have to cut out caffeine altogether, but you should cut back on it big time. Excessive caffeine consumption can increase the risk of miscarriage. Not to mention, caffeine is a diuretic . . . meaning it's going to make you have to pee a lot. What's more, it passes to breast milk, which can charge a breastfed baby's batteries. Sleep is good. We want sleep! A caffeinated baby sounds like a nightmare baby that defies gravity and crawls up walls. No new mommy wants that.

EXERCISE

If you are worried about having a lack of energy, think about the natural endorphins you could set into motion through some good old-fashioned exercise! Plus, fit moms are typically more ready for the intensity of labor. The key to exercising while pregnant is not to be a slug but not shoot for Olympic Gold, either. Be realistic, honest, and find a balance. Don't exercise to the point of being totally wiped out. If you have always led an active lifestyle, you should be able to continue your routine at a new pace that suits your current bod. If exercise was never your thing, don't think you need to start some crazy new workout regime as a pregnant warrior. Instead, take it slow and find a safe way to get your sweat on. Think about taking an afternoon walk or going for a casual swim in a pool. Riding a stationary bike is also a good bet, and plenty of yoga studios offer prenatal yoga.

It's also important to consider that some habits you might have had prior to becoming pregnant are no longer a good idea. For example, you want to avoid raising your body temperature too high. So, hot yoga, saunas, steam rooms, and aerobic exercise that sends your temp and heartbeat skyrocketing should take a backseat to cooler alternatives until your little guy or girl is out of the womb. This is your chance to chill out, hot mama! No need to sweat too much, you've got that prenatal sparkle and it's fabulous.

Pregnancy Journal

I am in love with:

_____

_____

_____

_____

I am always craving:

_____

_____

_____

_____

I am grossed out by:

_____

_____

_____

_____

I wonder if:

_____

_____

_____

_____

As a new Supermom, I vow to:

_____

_____

_____

_____

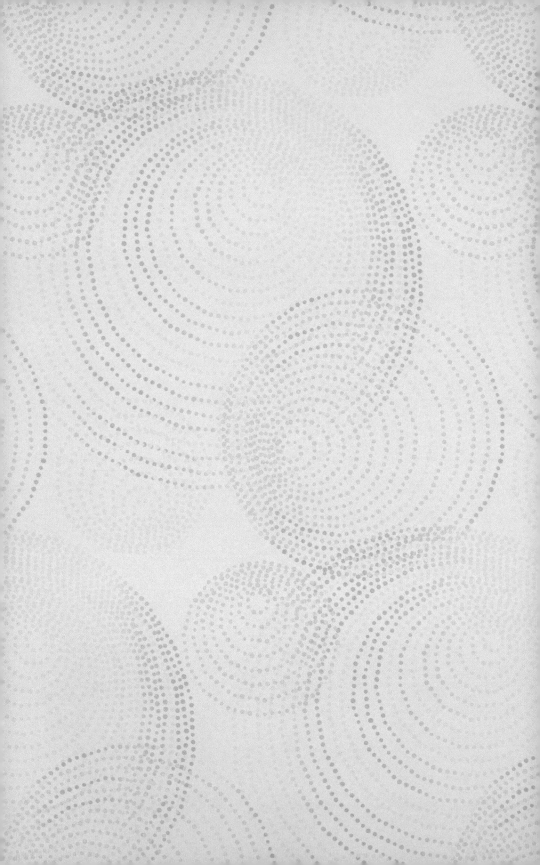

Chapter 3

PICKLES AND ICE CREAM

Milk products, fruit, chocolate, and salty snacks are the most common cravings of a pregnant woman, but don't let that stop your imagination from running wild. You do you, girlfriend. So is it mind over body or the other way around? The cravings you experience might possibly be hormone related. We blame everything else on hormones, so why not our hankering for pickles and ice cream? What does it mean if we want applesauce or sauerkraut instead? Could cravings be connected to our increased need for calories when we are pregnant? If we have cravings for chocolate and random stuff at various stages of our menstrual cycle, the same could be said for pregnancy. That's our story and we're sticking to it. Silly hormones and their peer pressure to scarf down all things delicious!

BODIES KNOW BETTER

There's some debate about whether or not our bodies are telling us we need something when we crave certain foods. Some think that craving a tall glass of milk might point to a need for calcium. Feeling a strong desire for certain types of fruits might mean you need more Vitamin C in your life. Some even believe that a shortage of magnesium can trigger a craving for chocolate. Yeah, that's it. Magnesium. Except, other foods that contain magnesium are composed of whole grains, beans, nuts, and vegetables. Are we craving all of those things covered in chocolate, maybe?

> "I craved meatballs and peaches. . . . Random! Not at the same time, but I definitely ate at least four peaches a day!"
>
> —*Casey*

SMART MINDS KNOW BEST

Some researchers are tired of hearing all these excuses to binge on random cravings and argue that nutritional needs have nothing to do with it. Instead, they insist we are looking for reasons to consume something we enjoy. What a bunch of party poopers! They suggest we desire particular foods based on what we think they signify. As if we might subconsciously start to crave something salty or sweet based on whether we want a boy or girl. These Debby Downers support their buzzkill (though potentially accurate) claims by saying that a woman typically doesn't crave anything that is a go-to source for the nutritional element her body is lacking. Instead, we crave specific foods, like delicious French fries. Okay, maybe these fries aren't serving a dietary purpose, but they are scrumptious!

It's no surprise that cravings can be culturally influenced. We crave what we know, so a girl in Thailand might have different cravings than a girl in America, and vice versa. What's more, there are some cases where women crave what they don't know. It's hard to picture how one might be able to do that, but there is a condition called Pica in which pregnant women crave odd items that are inedible on any other given day.

PECULIAR MUD PIES

Pica is Latin for magpie, a bird that is notorious for eating basically anything and everything, like a former high school wrestler. It may as well be Latin for mud pie, because chances are if you experience Pica, you will be fixing one up in the backyard and eating it for breakfast. Important: please do not indulge in mud pies and non-foods like paint chips.

Some women might crave laundry detergent, clay, or just plain dirt. This can be an indicator that they might be deficient in a particular nutrient like iron or zinc. Do not eat or drink toxic things. Even if the idea of it somehow sounds enticing, step away from the laundry detergent—and maybe even the laundry. Play the pregnancy card and get someone else to do the wash. Call your doctor at once if you are experiencing any of these kooky urges to consume something that isn't meant to be consumed. That's the serious part.

Now, let's play around with the concept of exploring what real food cravings might mean so that you can predict your baby's gender!

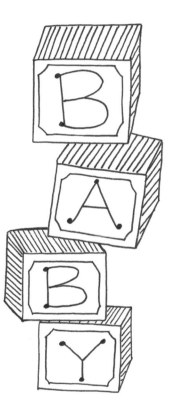

OLD WIVES' TALES AND SUPERSTITIONS

Who doesn't like a good old game of *Guess Who*? Does your baby have hair? Will your baby wear glasses? Before science stepped in to tell women how to do this and how not to do that, old wives were the head honchos in the jibber-jabber of baby care. Let's remember something about old ladies and grandmothers: They are typically stubborn and they aren't always right! Or, somehow, they are always right and know just what to do in every crisis. That wisdom, it wasn't born yesterday. The origin of "old wives' tales" traces back to 300 BC. While the baby's sex is determined at the time of fertilization by the type of sperm that fertilizes the egg, there's a bunch of ways to guess whether that baby is a boy or girl along the way. These might not be accurate guesses, but why should that stop us from having fun?

> "The old wives' tale I remember the most was that you shouldn't hang clothes outside on a clothesline because the wind might jerk the line out of your hand and could cause you to have a miscarriage."
>
> —*Judy*

BOY OR GIRL?

Are scientists as wise as old wives? Just ask your grandmother. Actually, she might tell you that if you pick up your keys from the long end, you're having a boy, and if you pick them up from the short end, you're having a girl. If you have baby brain, chances are you'll be lucky if you can even find your keys. Oops!

CRAVINGS

Are you worried that ignoring your cravings will give your baby a birthmark in the shape of the food you are craving? Some cultures believe that failing to cater to your cravings will leave a lasting imprint on your baby's skin. This is all likely mumbo jumbo, but why take a chance when your husband is ready and willing to go to the 24-hour supermarket to get you some Doritos at midnight? Why take a chance?!

SUGAR AND SPICE AND EVERYTHING DELICIOUS

Hey, cupcake. Does a spoonful of sugar help everything go down? If you can't get enough of the sweet stuff and you're all about eating those healthy fruits on top of a gallon of ice cream or inside a delicious pie, you might be having a girl. If you can eat a lot of garlic and not smell like it, congratulations! You aren't a vampire and you're still having a girl. Before you jump to that conclusion maybe kiss your partner and ask for a second opinion. Is your partner doing the whole sympathy weight-gain thing? That's sweet, as sweet as the cookies you've been craving because you're probably having a girl!

SPRINKLE THAT SALT

Are you a meat and potatoes kind of pregnant girl, instead? If you're grabbing pretzels, chips, and everything salty, you might be having a boy. If you're constantly bound for the meat counter and you're always craving burgers, fish, cheese, dairy, and basically a Hungry Man breakfast at all hours, the little boy inside of you is beginning to flex his manly appetite. It's also said that moms carrying boys crave more food each day in general, so get ready to eat like a football player.

BURNING LOVE

Craving hot sauce? Spice is nice, but go easy on the stuff. It won't make your baby blind (as some worry) but it may give you indigestion. Speaking of heartburn, if you experience a lot of it during pregnancy, you might be having a baby with a lot of hair! There's no solid proof that he'll come down the birth canal looking like Elvis, though. A hunk a hunk of burning love, that labor!

BLAME SCIENCE

Here's a star for science! Studies have shown that the foods and drinks a mommy ingests while pregnant can influence her baby's palate later in life. The flavors you consume also flavor the amniotic fluid that your baby starts swallowing in the second trimester. There's some support to the idea that a pregnant mom with a sweet tooth can pass it on to her baby. Meanwhile, eating vegetables while pregnant may help a baby develop a taste for them once they begin eating solid foods. Isn't that something? So, when your kids have zero interest in finishing their carrots, your secret of not eating them while pregnant is safe with us.

HEY, GOOD-LOOKING

Is your face rounder than usual? You might be having a girl. If it's slimmer and you're feeling svelte, you might be having a boy. If you're just bloated and feeling swollen on the inside, you're pregnant, and we already know that.

Oh, that pregnancy glow! If you have a bright complexion and your hair looks like it's moving in slow motion even when you're rushing out the door, you're probably having a boy. On the contrary, if your skin is breaking out and your hair is thinning, blame it on the little girl growing inside of you. People say she is likely to suck up all of your good looks! Well, at least you can hold onto your sanity until she becomes a teenager.

BABY BUMP BUSINESS

Some believe that if a woman is carrying her weight out front like a basketball, she is having a boy. If she is carrying her weight all over like a watermelon, she's having a girl. If you are carrying the baby low, it's a boy. If you are carrying the baby high, it's a girl. If you can still get down with your bad self, you're awesome and you're on your way to being a dance mom.

POTTY TRAINING

If your pee is bright yellow, you might be having a girl. If it's dull yellow, you might be having a boy. All of this could also mean you are a little dehydrated and should drink more water.

Feel like doing a science experiment and peeing in a cup? Who doesn't? Apparently, the baking soda test can help you figure out if you're having a boy or a girl. If you pee in the cup and it fizzes, it's a boy. If it stays flat, it's a girl. For heaven's sake, just don't drink it.

HOT WATER

Some pregnant women worry that taking a bath can be harmful to their baby. Taking a bath isn't going to drown your baby; in fact, it might give the little guy or girl a relaxing experience! Just be careful about how hot the temperature is. Avoid hot tubs and saunas. Water temperatures shouldn't exceed 98 degrees Fahrenheit. Listening to a 98 Degrees throwback CD while enjoying a lukewarm bubble bath never hurt anybody, though.

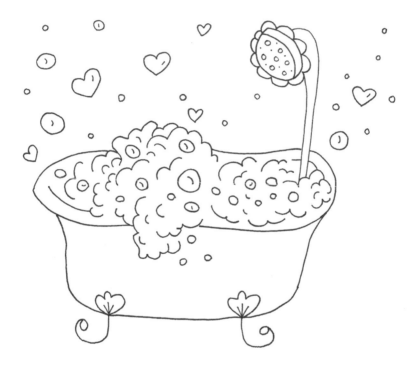

THE MOON

The Aztecs warned pregnant moms that looking at a lunar eclipse while they were expecting a child would lead the baby to develop a cleft lip. To protect herself and her baby, a mom should carry something metallic in her underwear, like a safety pin. Do rose gold panties count? They are awfully cute and an unhooked safety pin is a hoo-ha hazard.

MOVE THAT BABY

Pregnant moms are often asking if lifting your arms above your head will strangle your baby. It's a good excuse to ask people to retrieve things from high shelves, but raising your arms isn't going to make the umbilical cord strangle your baby in the womb. Thank goodness—how else would we blow dry our bangs?

Something else to think about: After sixteen weeks of being pregnant, you shouldn't lie on your back while exercising. This can decrease blood flow to the uterus and placenta, so those ten-minute ab workouts will have to wait. Gosh darn it!

Mommy's Letter to Baby

Pregnancy can be hard—but imagining the new relationship you're about to build with your child makes it all worth it. Let this page be a reminder of your hopes and dreams as a new mom. Is there anything you'd like your baby to know about this special time? What do you wish for your baby as they enter the world? What kind of mom do you promise to be?

Pregnancy Journal

I think I am having a:

_____

_____

_____

_____

Thank goodness for:

_____

_____

_____

_____

I really need:

_____

_____

_____

_____

I will never:

_____

_____

_____

_____

I will always:

_____

_____

_____

_____

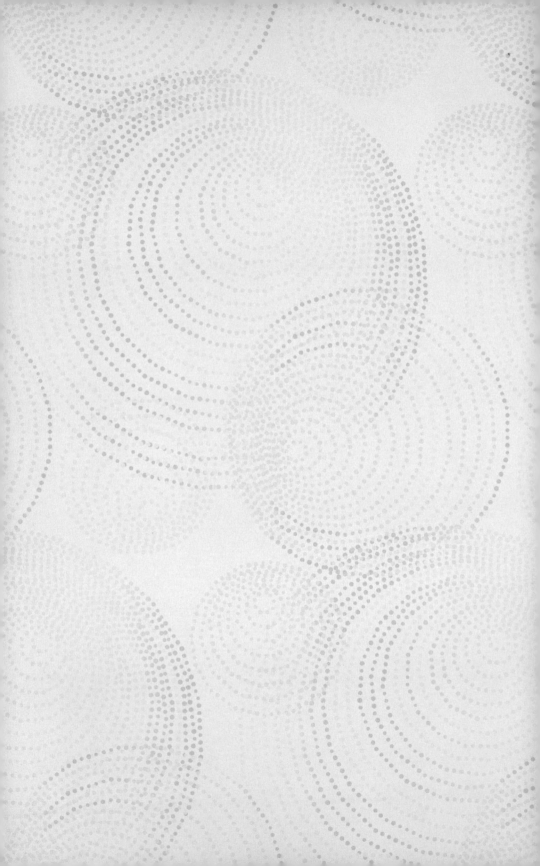

Chapter 4

CELEBRATING MOM AND BABY

In spite of the fun people have cutting into a pink cake to signify a baby girl's arrival or poking a clear balloon that sends blue confetti flying into the air to indicate a boy is on the way, it's interesting to consider that these two colors were once not indicative of either gender. Today, it's a natural response when decorating for a baby shower. If it's a girl, it's all pretty in pink! If it's a boy, it's cool blue all of the way, baby. Except, the two colors were not promoted as gender-specific until just before World War I. Marketing opportunists realized they could convince new moms they needed to buy an entirely new wardrobe for the second child if he or she had a sister or brother by suggesting different colors for each. That's because pastels were all the rage when they were introduced in the mid-nineteenth century, but before anyone was even considering filling their closets with colorful fabrics, for centuries boys and girls both donned little white dresses until they were about six or seven years old. It's said that white was a popular baby dress choice because it was easier to bleach and keep clean. Honestly, how does that really make sense? White clothes are essentially destined to be dirtied by any type of red food additive or unfortunate bodily malfunction—everyone knows that—and what sane mom wants a bland wash-and-fold headache? Moms aren't crazy, they're celebrated every year thanks to one eccentric lady committed to honoring her own mother's memory.

Mothers and babies alike have long been showered and honored in a variety of ways that have grown over time, but one thing is certain. Despite the societal norms that sometimes give moms a hard time, the miracle of child birth has always been cherished by the communities that surround the dynamic duo of mother and child.

THE BABY SHOWER

Perhaps one of the most anticipated and exciting events of a woman's first pregnancy is her baby shower, when she and her baby are showered with gifts and love. There are games, glam, and so many smiles throughout the day as a close-knit community celebrates the anticipated arrival of a little button of a person. How cute! This fun part of becoming a new mom hasn't always taken the shape of big bows and pastel balloons, but gatherings of people have long been honoring moms as they bring new life into the world.

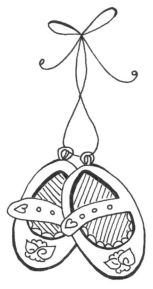

ANCIENT ROME, GREECE, AND EGYPT

The Ancient Greeks and Romans kept pregnant women confined before and just after birth. How lonely! If smart phones were around then, would these isolated women have been taking mirror selfies to keep every distant relative in the loop? Probably not, because everyone thought the process of pregnancy was a little too dirty to be seen or talked about. Mommies-to-be were sequestered like they had the plague while gladiators were saluted on center stage. How sweet!

Moms and their babies were welcomed back into society after they were all cleaned up and purified, perhaps as an apology for being chastised like criminals or contagious patients. It's during these festivals and post-birth fun times that the baby was formally named. Similarly, Ancient Egyptians preferred to celebrate after the baby was born, when both mom and baby were purified. Pregnancy, how dare it be so dirty!

MIDDLE AGES

During the Middle Ages, the mom was hidden away for a month and a half following the birth of her baby. The main birth celebration held between the fifth and fifteenth centuries was all about God, as the Christian baptism became the go-to way to honor and bless new life. Godparents played a crucial role in this religious event and would honor the newborn baby with a special token or gift. It didn't take long for smart aleck parents to realize that requesting more godparents meant getting more gifts. As a result, the church had to limit the number of godparents a family could name to make sure the relationship wasn't tainted by greed. Since then, babies have relied on aunts and uncles to make up the difference.

VICTORIAN ERA

Pregnant women still weren't quite fit to be seen in public during the Victorian Era, as it was considered poor manners. How dare a big belly grace the sunlight? To the shadows a mommy-to-be went until it was time to be showered with gifts. New moms joined in celebrating with other ladies at a frilly tea party after the whole nasty childbirth business was over. Women played fun pregnancy games and romanticized over how cute that little nugget baby turned out to be in spite of the gross pregnancy part. If it was the mother's second pregnancy, she'd be sprinkled with gifts because she didn't need as much new stuff and wasn't as icky the second time around.

MODERN-DAY BABY SHOWERS

The baby shower as we know it today began building in the early 1900s and really took shape during the baby boom era just after World War II. These celebrations started with one core purpose: to help support new couples with their financial and practical needs as they welcomed new life into the world. Since then, baby showers have become a happy gathering to not only support the celebration of childbirth but also the beauty in being pregnant.

Pregnant moms are no longer hiding in closets and faraway nooks. Today, they are going to work, getting outside, and parking in spots designated just for them. They are proving that pregnancy should earn a woman a first-row seat, not a backstage hideaway. Your baby bump is beautiful, darling. Thankfully, modern society agrees!

Top 10 Baby Shower Songs

"Baby Love" by The Supremes

"There Goes My Baby" by The Drifters

"Be My Baby" by The Ronettes

"Don't Worry Baby" by The Beach Boys

"Sweet Child O' Mine" by Guns N' Roses

"I Got You Babe" by Sonny and Cher

"I Knew I Loved You" by Savage Garden

"I'll Stand by You" by The Pretenders

"Baby, I Love Your Way" by Peter Frampton

"Everything I Do" by Bryan Adams

Mommy's Baby Registry Ideas

Some popular registry items include a sleeper or bassinet, diapers and diaper pail, sound machine, car seat, stroller, baby wrap and/or carrier, adorable baby clothes, bibs and/or burp cloths, breast pump and/or formula with a bottle drying rack, baby nasal aspirator, baby wipe warmer, and a booster seat.

MOTHER'S DAY

Moms should have two holidays: Mother's Day and Labor Day. Labor Day was first introduced in 1882, and mothers had been giving birth and working hard long before then! So, it's no surprise that Mother's Day cards are one of the highest holiday greeting card sellers just behind Christmas and Valentine's Day. Watching our babies grow to surprise us, impress us, and make us proud are the greatest daily gifts we could receive. Flowers and cards couldn't hurt though, right? Well, the woman credited with founding Mother's Day in the United States, Anna Jarvis, had plenty of bones to pick with the commercialized business of the holiday.

> "My mom always hugged us and told us everything would be alright,
> no matter how big or small the problem was."
> —*Christy*

THE MOTHER OF MOTHER'S DAY

Mother's Day was inspired by Anna Jarvis, who wanted to honor her own mother, Anne Reeves Jarvis, who in the 1850s pioneered work clubs to help educate new moms and lower infant mortality rates. Her groups also helped wounded soldiers from both the North and the South during the Civil War. When Mama Jarvis passed away in 1905, her daughter Anna was determined to do something to pay homage to moms everywhere. She first celebrated Mother's Day in 1908 and was so driven by her dedication to moms that in 1914, President Woodrow Wilson officially set aside the second Sunday in May for everyone to celebrate and honor their mothers.

PURE INTENTIONS

Anna Jarvis's intention of honoring moms was grand, as was her pride, and she took great pride in being the founder of Mother's Day. Her mom's favorite flower, the white carnation, was the original flower of the holiday. When everyone began to paint the day with their own pastels, Anna Jarvis became dissatisfied with the marketing. One can empathize with the good-intentioned girl who became a bitter woman. Her heart was pure even if it was stubborn. Still, we can all agree with her that moms should be honored. Ideally, we should try to let our own moms know how much we appreciate them regularly and not just on a calendar date.

"My mom said, 'No matter what, I'll never judge you.' This was especially important during my teen years when I was getting into trouble. I was rebellious and yet uncertain in the world. I knew that I could call her anytime and she would be there."
–*Caitlin*

CELEBRATING THE WORLD'S GREATEST MOM

So, how does one begin to verbalize how to thank a Supermom? How do you celebrate your own mother each year? Are flowers and cards a necessary piece of the thankful pie? Sometimes, it's hard to find the words. Flowers and cards are nice, but the important thing is that we ourselves recognize, more than once a year, just what being a mother means to our little ones and the rest of the world. Golly, we *are* the greatest!

Pregnancy Journal

My baby shower was:

_____

_____

_____

_____

My favorite moment was:

_____

_____

_____

_____

I will always cherish:

_____

_____

_____

_____

Mother's Day will be:

_____

_____

_____

_____

_____

I want my baby to know that:

_____

_____

_____

_____

_____

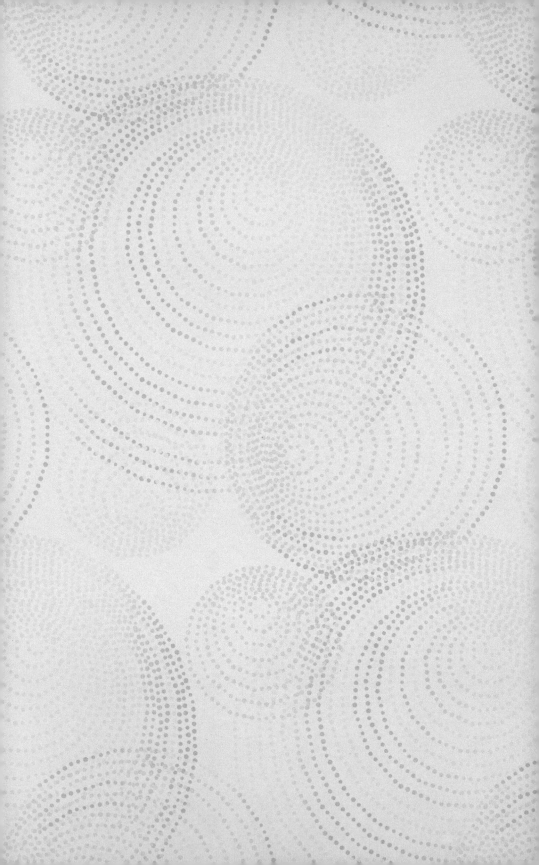

Chapter 5

THE WORLD'S GREATEST HONOR

Becoming a mom might very well be the most important, impressive, and lasting thing a woman does in life. Not every woman is destined for motherhood, and that's totally fine, but the ladies who do have this role carved into their lifelines deserve a medal, a raise, or at the very least a pat on the back—preferably a massage. Moms don't have sick time guaranteed into their work schedule, they don't earn a dime, and they hardly take any personal days off. Instead, they are perpetually exhausted, they trade in their shoe budget for baby care, and replace the pampering of their fingernails with the Pampers™ required for their little tykes. For this reason, it's so important to realize, recognize, and remember that mommies matter too.

INSPIRING WOMEN

Mommies fix the bad stuff, kiss the bruises, and make everything else better. This devotion is programmed into their wiring! Moms weren't created to serve us, they created us. We owe them our very existence. *Gasp!* Perhaps the most inspiring thing about moms is their charming ability to multitask without their kids realizing they have other priorities to manage. How did our mothers know how to handle every situation? Chances are, they never actually carried all of the knowledge in the world, but they do still carry the guilt of that one time they forgot to pack us lunch. This baggage moms lug around is the baby weight we'll never lose, except, we'll learn to cope with our decisions by realizing our kids will understand in time. When they need a hug, we'll be there to squeeze them tight. When they need a

> "When I was in elementary school, my mom worked evening shifts a few nights a week as a nurse, so she couldn't always be home to greet me. On those occasions, she would leave scavenger hunts at the house for us, with fun clues and small little treats at the end. It was such a simple and small thing, but I loved the excitement of those days!"
>
> *—Jenny*

push in the right direction, we'll be the ones offering them a metaphorical kick in the rear.

ALWAYS A MOM

As we enter into a new chapter of our lives as new moms, our own mothers are stepping into new roles as grandmothers. This precious transition helps us understand one another better, and we need that mother-daughter friendship more than ever.

> "One of the most important things my mother did for me was to be both a friend and a mom. I knew my mother would always be there for me whenever and wherever I needed her. I always tried to do the same with my children."
>
> *—Judy*

GUIDING THE FUTURE

Motherhood may not be about living vicariously through the successes of little leaguers and softball sluggers, but there's no harm in taking pride in a child's triumphs. We can't always know what is best for our kids. We can only hope that we teach them how to decipher those really tough decisions for themselves. We give them the guidance, the love, and the name. Their future careers and lives are up to them.

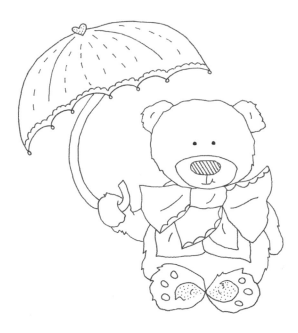

"One of the most important things my mother did for me was to show me that she cared, but she also disciplined me. She didn't let me get away with much, yet supported me in all that I did. She gave me the proper balance that I needed to be a productive adult."

— *Casey*

When looking at the lives of successful men and women, we would be naïve to not consider the impact their parents had on their achievement. People shouldn't blame their parents for everything, but they can credit them with at least half of the good stuff. Being a mom means being criticized for what went wrong and being heralded for what went right. It's a wrenching push-and-pull on the heart strings, and it's not an easy ride. But it's the greatest honor in the world.

Mommy's Letter to Grandma

What is the one of the most important things your mother did for you as a child that you would hope to continue to do for your own child? Is there anything you would like your baby's grandmother to know? Share a favorite memory you experienced with your mom or write down a wish you have for her as she takes on a new role as a grandmother.

_____

_____

_____

_____

_____

_____

_____

_____

_____

_____

_____

_____

_____

_____

_____

_____

_____

_____

_____

_____

_____

CREATING LEADERS

Could the successes of a person be traced back
to the close or nonexistent relationship they had
with their mother? There's something to be said
about mama's boys. The phrase has a conde-
scending feel to it, but its meaning reflects a
man's lifelong attachment to his mother. What's
so wrong with a guy letting his mother know
just how much she means to him? Obviously,
a mother-son relationship evolves and a mom

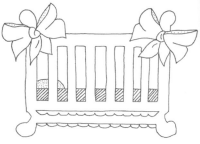

isn't going to be the same figure to a grown man as she was to him as a child. Her
tone may change, but she will always be mom. That's important.

UNITED STATES PRESIDENTS

Old presidents had a stoic exterior, but it turns out many of them were a bunch of
softies with a serious love for their mommies! Who could blame them for wanting
to keep their hearts close to home once setting up shop in the Oval Office? Mothers always know just what to do, and there's no harm in resorting back to a love
they could lean on when the entire country was counting on these guys to do right
by their jobs as president.

THOMAS WOODROW WILSON

It's no coincidence that the man who made Mother's Day official had a lifelong
love and admiration for his own mother, Jessie Woodrow Wilson. Before the world
knew (Thomas) Woodrow Wilson as the 28th United States President, he was
just Tommy to his mommy. They both agreed that Woodrow sounded much more
stately for a grown man, and so Thomas came to honor his mother's maiden name
for life. She continued to inspire her son's commitment to treating women with
respect and advocating for world peace.

TRUMAN LOVE

Harry Truman called his mom, Martha Young Truman, from the oval office once or
twice per week. He and his wife frequently went to his mother's house for Sunday

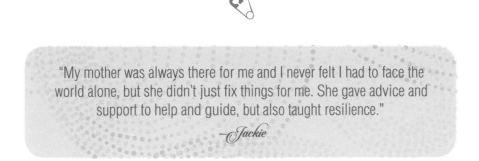

dinner early on in their marriage and mama dukes would sit on platforms with Harry to provide advice. He wrote her letters often and had a portrait of good old mom hanging in the white house! When her son hit the big time at 1600 Pennsylvania Avenue, his down-to-Earth mama remained humble but proud. Her son wasn't the only top dog that penned his mother on the regular. Eisenhower wrote his mom a bunch too! They'd probably be even closer now in the digital age. Could you picture the 34th American president sending happy face emojis to his mommy?

FOREVER A SON

William Harding was known for sending his dear mom flowers on Sunday, and Lyndon Johnson was not shy about calling his mother the greatest woman he ever knew. He had no quips about giving her a call to get her opinion when in the middle of a meeting, either. Teaching him the alphabet before he was two years old really stuck with him for life. Calvin Coolidge lost his mother when he was only twelve years old. It's said that he died with a picture of her in an old watch that was hanging over his heart. No matter where life takes them, mothers are always close to their children's hearts, that's for sure.

MOMS ON A MISSION

You don't have to be the mother of a president to make a difference or prove your worth. Since the dawn of time, mothers have graced the world with the accomplishments of their children, but likewise with their own personal goals as women on a mission. It's like moms are gifted with a double whammy, in a good way. Now, you don't just have the chance to go after your own dreams; you can also facilitate the dreams of your kids.

THE FLYING HOUSEWIFE

Need inspiration to get your body back in gear after giving birth? When you're feeling lazy, you might want to think about Fanny Blankers Koen, also known as the Flying Housewife. This impressive mother of two was pregnant with her third child when she won four gold medals at the 1948 Summer Olympics in London. She was later named the International Association of Athletics Federations (IAAF) Female Athlete of the 20th Century in 1999!

PHYSICS OF PARENTING

Feeling tired of baby brain and need some motivation to get your head back on straight? Let your thoughts be inspired by Marie Curie. She wasn't just the first woman to win the Nobel Prize as a legit physicist. She dug deep to find a balance after her husband was killed in an accident and went on to raise their two beautiful daughters on her own. One of those girls would go on to follow in Mommy's footsteps by winning a Nobel prize in chemistry with her own husband too!

BEING A MOM COUNTS

Ada Lovelace was a mathematician and the first computer programmer in the world, and her most impactful work was completed while she was balancing life as a mom. And let's not forget Sojourner Truth, who escaped slavery with her baby daughter in 1826 to learn that her five-year-old son had been illegally sold to some guy in Alabama. Determined, Truth raised money to get her son back by successfully suing a white man in court. Talk about resilience!

INSPIRING OUR BEST

Children help us find new inspiration for devoting our time to important ventures. Think about Jessica Alba, an actress who became a mother and successful businesswoman. Alba founded *The Honest Company* because she was searching for household and baby products that were free from harmful chemicals.

> "Being a mom is *everything* to me. My girls are my reason.
> They make me laugh, cry, frustrate me, and feel every emotion
> there is . . . but there is nothing better than being a mom."
> —*Casey*

If you think having children is going to change your life, you are right. Children might put a fork in the road in terms of your pre-mommy plans, but chances are the redirection will fuel you toward something better. Let stories of successful moms inspire you, not intimidate you. You are going to define your own greatness. You don't have to make other people's history books to matter or to prove your worth. Your family history is the story that counts. Be you—you are already amazing—and your story will leave an imprint in the hearts of your children.

> "My mother did so much for us when we were kids. She never put
> herself before us. She is one of the most selfless people I know and I
> hope that I show my kids the same love that my mom showed us."
> —*Kate*

Pregnancy Journal

I promise to:

_____

_____

_____

_____

_____

I really admire:

_____

_____

_____

_____

_____

If I need help, I can depend on:

_____

_____

_____

_____

_____

I think my baby will be the next:

_____

_____

_____

_____

No matter what, I want my child to be:

_____

_____

_____

_____

_____

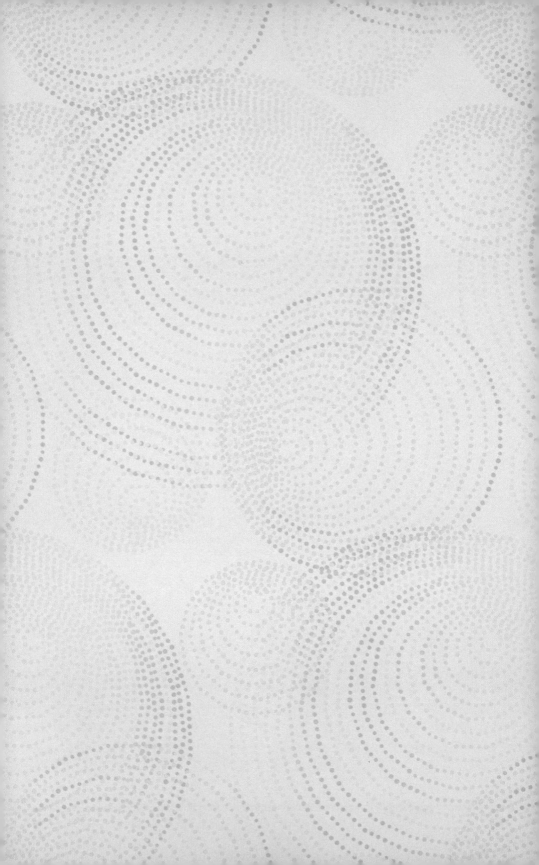

Chapter 6

MOMMY NATURE

It's no coincidence and seemingly only natural that nature has long been personified as a woman. Not only a woman, but a mother that gives birth to life. Mother Nature is known to be temperamental with her violent displays of tumultuous wreckage, sometimes experienced firsthand and many times explained through secondhand, word-of-mouth reports from meteorologists, many of whom are never able to figure this worldly female out or predict her next move! Sometimes, Mother Nature simply can't decide what she's in the mood for, rain or snow? Will she be hot or cold today? Is she sitting at a perpetual restaurant table contemplating the weather menu? Does she want a little bit of what Father Time is having?

PREDICTING PREGNANT WIVES

Navigating the path of the hormonal tornado that's taking shape in a woman's pregnant body is no simple challenge. We can learn a great deal from the big lady that runs the outdoor show. Mother Nature can be stern, but she is soft too.

Flowers bloom in the spring. Hair grows back (unless you are a man of a certain age, and definitely if you are a woman of a certain age—what's up with those chin hairs, anyway?). The sun is there to warm us after a threatening storm, and it keeps rising every day, even after it burns us on the beach. In a way, that's what being a mom might be all about. Getting up and figuring it out, every day, rising like the sun.

Will we instinctively know just what to do with our own little munchkins? Somehow, it's certain we will be fine. There's the nature aspect of mothering, which we also see in animal moms. We can't forget about the nurture, though. The love our own moms gave us definitely taught us a lot.

THE ANIMAL QUEENDOM

Moms of the animal world are bosses, so why is it called a kingdom? Science has shown us more than just what's happening in our own bodies. We have gained a great deal of knowledge about how mothers in the animal kingdom care for their young. It's pretty empowering knowing that there are moms out there, just like us, making life happen. What better way to gain inspiration for our own pregnant strife and success than to realize we're not the only big mamas doing our part to keep the world afloat? As it turns out, human moms aren't the only beings that have a hard time letting go of their little ones, and we aren't the only ones willing to do whatever we can to protect our kids.

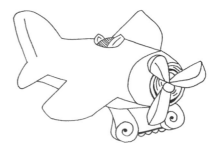

BIRD MOMS

Ospreys are the reality show moms that thrive on drama to take care of their little ones. These birds are committed to protecting their nests at all costs, and they have to have the last word. Sounds like a typical chick! Speaking of drama, the next time someone calls you cuckoo, you should take offense. (Here's a tip for what *not* to do as a mom.) Cuckoo birds are essentially the worst of the bad bird moms. They squat in other birds' nests, then leave their own eggs there on the doorstep! What's worse, the cuckoo babies are typically bigger than the other chicks in the nest, so when they hatch, they force the smaller birds out of their own home! Meanwhile, the cuckoo mama has already moved on to the next flavor of the week on the roof of some local pub, totally ignoring her responsibilities as a mama bird. For humans, a much better option would be to make friends with the neighboring mom in order to exchange rotisserie chicken recipes over a bottle of wine.

SEA MOMS

There are plenty of fish in the sea, and they're all being homeschooled. Bottlenose dolphin moms are all about creating a cute little passive-aggressive leash to keep their kids in check. It's for their own safety and development! The little babes swim near the moms and nobody has to worry about them getting lost on the trip because of the hydrodynamic wake mamas build to keep their young nearby. How genius!

HOME FOR DINNER

Who knew that salmon were so sentimental? Salmon moms swim their way back to the waters where they were first born in order to reproduce. A female salmon will dig a hole in her homeland gravel, then lay her eggs there, leaving them fresh for a salmon dude to come along and fertilize the bunch. These babies start out their lives living under rocks, then hit the current of the water once they have enough strength and confidence. That's where they continue to grow, and from there they make their way off to sea. When the girls get the urge to reproduce, they don't just lay their eggs anywhere like a lazy Sally. Instead, they embark on an arduous expedition upstream to return home.

RIP OCTOMOMS

The giant Pacific octopus is seriously legit when it comes to caring for her babies, and she is willing to pay the ultimate sacrifice. Her destiny is to have one successful collection of offspring in her lifetime—that means, like two hundred thousand baby eggs. No big deal, though! After months and months of holding the same yoga pose over her eggs to keep them protected, warm, oxygenated, and free of yucky bacteria things, the octopus gives life to the little squirts by sending them out into the ocean using muscular organs called siphons. Once that happens, the mom typically dies from exhaustion or starvation. She just doesn't have the energy to fight back against shameless predator types eager to capitalize on her weak condition. Let's now take a moment to mentally send every octomom in existence our thoughts, prayers, and respect.

EMPEROR PENGUINS

If we're handing out animal superlatives, emperor penguins are definitely the cutest couple. The mom lays her egg, trusts the dad to watch over and protect it for months, then departs on a journey of up to fifty miles in search of food. No gender barriers here—the mom and dad are working as a team to keep their baby alive, and they're just adorable, right?

DEADBEAT ANIMAL DADS

Not all animal dads are stand-up dudes. Male and female cheetahs, for instance, only hang out to mate. A cheetah mom can have up to nine cubs at a time. The responsibility-free dad basically ditches the family and immediately goes off on his own while the mom is left to raise and train the little ones all by herself. The cubs are born blind with zero survival skills, so the mom puts on her favorite 1980s rock song playlist and workout sneakers, then gets to work by bringing home prey for the kiddos to practice on and learn from. Cue the training montage!

BRR! THAT'S COLD, DAD

Maybe cheetah dads are out grabbing a beer with polar bear dads, since polar bear moms are also on their own when it comes to raising their kin. Pregnant polar bears dig an underground den to keep warm from super cold temperatures. They go into hibernation and give birth between November and February. The moms fast for eight months but need to gain at least double their body weight, which is a mere four hundred pounds. Otherwise—get this—their bodies will absorb the fetuses. Why these poor polar bear moms don't have their own reality show is still a mystery.

MOMS WITH A MOUTH

Alligator moms are such big softies! They lay thirty to fifty eggs and then carry their babies around in their mouths. It's like when your family has an enormous, vicious dog that is really just a teddy bear when other people aren't around. In fact, you would even feel safe sticking your hand in his mouth to retrieve a sock he stole from your drawer.

CUTE AND ICKY

Everyone knows koalas are all about that eucalyptus plant. However, the plant leaves are poisonous suckers and the koalas need to build up their tolerance to digest them. Big koalas already have that in play but the babies need to develop this function. So, what's an animal mom to do but eat her own feces and feed it to her young? Yum. That way, the babies get the broken down version of the real deal and can learn to catch up. They probably all have pinkeye, but that's a small price to pay. As marsupials are born without fur, ears, or eyes, maybe that's how they get away with it.

STRONG AND ITSY-BITSY

Wolf spiders carry their eggs and baby spiders on their backs until the tiny, eight-legged tykes are old enough to care for themselves. There's a stern understanding that they won't be freeloaders playing video games all day, though.

SWEET SIXTEEN

If your pregnancy feels like a long time, know that elephant moms carry their babies for twenty-two months! They also have the biggest babies, weighing in at around 200–250 pounds. It's so cute though, because other female elephants in the herd help babysit and take care of the babies. Born blind, the little elephant babies have to rely on their mommy's trunk to navigate the world at first. Maybe that's why they stick with their mothers for up to sixteen years. Then, the herd throws the adolescent elephant an epic sweet sixteen birthday party with the entire animal kingdom there.

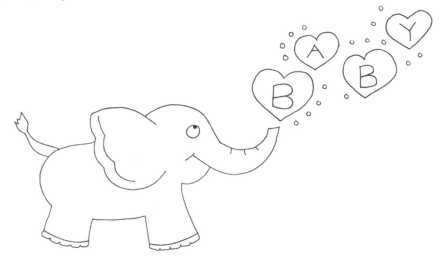

SMART MOMS

Orangutans have babies every eight years or so and breastfeed them until they are five years old. Maybe it's the 97 percent of the human DNA orangutans share with us that makes them forge a lasting relationship with their kin. Or, maybe we're the reason they have the neurotic behavior of building a brand-new nest every night. Actually, that sounds like a lot of work! Orangutans build thousands of homes in their lifetime. Talk about real estate!

"You will always be the one they call on or need. When you least expect it or are having a bad day and that little three-year-old says, 'I love you, Mommy,' those moments just put life's craziness into perspective. You can never say I love you too much."

—Christy

CATS

There's a rumor that cats have a natural urge to smother babies. This isn't true—they aren't plotting to hurt your little one (or are they? Depends on whether or not you are a cat person). Cats have a tendency to want to snuggle up next to something soft and warm, so a sleeping baby might just be the spot. Cats do pose an actual danger to pregnant ladies and their babies, though. Cat feces can carry a parasite that causes toxoplasmosis, which can be spread to humans. It's a pesky disease that infects multiple organs in the fetus and causes anything from deafness to respiratory problems. Yuck. Instead of taking a risk with changing the litter box, ask your partner to do you a solid this year. If you live alone and there is nobody else to change the litter box, wear gloves or be very careful with how you handle the stuff and always, always wash your hands. Like everything, double check with your doctor to decide your best option.

Pregnancy Journal

My spirit animal is:

_____
_____
_____
_____
_____

My body feels:

_____
_____
_____
_____
_____

My mind is:

_____
_____
_____
_____

I wish that:

_____

_____

_____

_____

_____

Chapter 7

THE MAGIC OF MOTHERHOOD

If animal moms seem like they know exactly what they are doing, maybe it's because they don't have the added pressure of society telling them how to do everything. They're just out there living their lives and letting nature's call guide them. Humans seem to know their place in the animal kingdom, but not quite in each other's conversations about how to be a good mom. When we don't have the threat of being eaten on a hiking trail, we stand high and mighty with our noses stretched up toward the sky. We are the best of the best here on Earth! Boy, we are magical. Even if we ourselves don't know the right way of doing something, we definitely know that our neighbor's way of doing something has to be wrong. Many of us are over here analyzing and overanalyzing. Meanwhile, some of us are just agonizing about our next steps. *Gulp.* How do we know that our way will be the right way?

Meanwhile, we don't look at animal moms and tell them they are doing it wrong (with the exception of the cuckoo bird, who is, well, cuckoo). We don't make them feel depressed because carrying a bunch of spiders on their backs seems like it might be a little excessive. We don't judge the meerkat when it teaches its babies how to catch and handle a scorpion. (*Gasp!* How dangerous is that?! Do the meerkat cubs even wear helmets?) Instead, we read about these impressive animal moms or simply observe them, in awe of their intelligence.

GOOD INTENTIONS GO A LONG WAY

Animal moms don't have financial pressure and they don't have bills. They are free of debt and they aren't consumed by the latest trends. They are an important constant to help us remember, motherhood has been a staple of life through the ages, long before pink and blue were fashionable. Through the years, human moms have gotten a lot of grief from outsiders about how they should raise their children. Since it changes so often, how do we know that what we are told today won't be the opposite tomorrow? How do we handle the uncertainty of change in

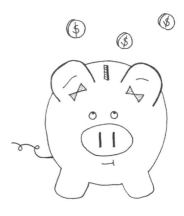

psychological opinions of how to parent? Will a doctor's advice actually push our child into therapy? Gosh, will everything be our fault? The answer is no, because every one of our own challenges is not all our mother's fault, either. When we act with the best intentions, we can release some of that mom guilt.

> "In my era you were fortunate to be able to enjoy your new baby. Many new moms had the luxury to be able to stay home and give their child their full attention. Today it's very stressful, I think, on new moms because not only are they experiencing this wonderful time in their lives, but because many if not all moms have to work outside the home to make ends meet."
>
> —Judy

TOUGH LOVE

In the early 1900s, "good" moms were all about being bad cops giving tough love. The fad was to handle babies as little as possible. This idea stuck around through the 1920s when experts advised mothers not to give their children too many snuggles. Otherwise, they might be enabling future criminals! Hugging and kissing your child to let them know you were human was a mistake. Be a robotic mom, instead! That maternal instinct to cuddle up with your kiddo? It was wrong. Walk away and let the cries commence, moms were often told.

ENOUGH LOVE

The cold advice from experts back then was a far cry from what some say is common practice more than a century later. What would moms of 1910 say about helicopter parenting and helping kids a little too much with their homework? *Gasp.* What's ruining future generations this decade? It's funny how the wheel turns and mothers continue to wipe away the puke from their shoulders, shrugging at what the next expert opinion concurs is best. So, how do we find the balance?

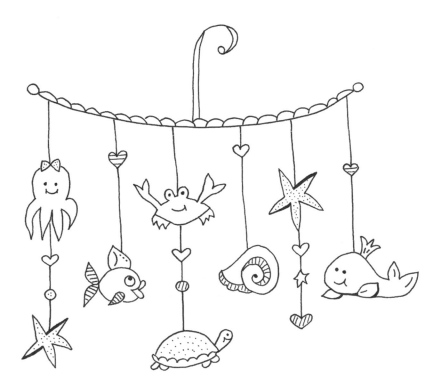

> "Don't stress. Babies can feel it."
>
> —*Jenny*

How does one define the word "expert"? Is it the psychologists reading about the theory of how the child's brain functions? Or is it the real moms out there on the front lines of parenting, witnessing and just knowing how their child's brain functions? Being told what works and experiencing what works firsthand are two different things. Perhaps we can learn a little bit from both.

> "Being a mom is the hardest job, both physically and mentally. But looking at my sons when they are happy definitely makes the job worth it. That and cuddle time!"
>
> —*Kate*

CUDDLE TIME

After decades of moms being told they were cruel humans if they weren't being strict with their kids, a new notion settled in and stuck around. Dr. Benjamin Spock broke the mold on motherhood and parenting with his book, *Baby & Child Care*, published in 1946. For the first time, mothers were told their instinct of wanting to love and nurture their babies was actually a good thing.

Whereas moms of the 1920s were told that giving too much affection to their kids would lead to criminal behavior, moms of the 1940s and 1950s were told children deprived of affection would suffer other kinds of emotional damage. So . . . moms were in trouble no matter what. Thank goodness for the free living of the 1970s when new moms threw up their arms in retreat. People realized that nobody needed to be an expert to be a good mom. Poof—the ridiculous pressure was gone, for a moment—then we realized we put pressure on ourselves too.

> "I was twenty-seven when I got pregnant with Peyton. I remember everyone being so critical of moms. I think it's changed since I had Peyton almost nine years ago, or maybe I just found that I don't care as much what other people think or say. I'm their mom, and I know what is best for me and my girls."
>
> *—Casey*

BE YOU

There's always going to be a mom that's better than you at something, and one that's worse than you at something else. That's how life works. You can always be better, but don't get down on yourself about that. You aren't the best, and you aren't the worst. You are you, and the most beautiful parts of you are currently growing into a little version of you as we speak!

PERSPECTIVE

It's all perspective, Mama. Does it seem like your coworker has all of her stuff together because she's constantly posting epic family pictures on social media? A filtered photo doesn't show that it was four o'clock in the afternoon when it was taken, and that she hadn't even brushed her teeth or eaten a smidge of food yet. The bags under her eyes were edited out. Chances are, every mom is out there just trying to make it through the day.

THE MANY WAYS OF MOTHERING

June Cleaver daintily cleaned in high heels, Kitty Foreman drank too much, and Roseanne Conner was crass and cunning. Becoming a mom isn't a character you're about to play in front of a critical audience. Don't worry about the peanut gallery or the neighbor's ratings because there is no one good way to mother. There's the path that's right for you, and that's what matters. Your way might not necessarily be right for the next mom, and that's okay too. Trust yourself. Being a parent is not about being a politician or a preacher. Being a mom means something different to everyone. It's good to be inspired by others, but let others be inspired by you too! Some are going to say a mom should spend a certain number of hours with her

Top 10 TV Moms

Carol Brady from *The Brady Bunch*

Claire Dunphy from *Modern Family*

Roseanne Conner from *Roseanne*

Marion Cunningham from *Happy Days*

Daenerys Targaryen from *Game of Thrones*

Peggy Bundy from *Married with Children*

June Cleaver from *Leave it to Beaver*

Kitty Foreman from *That 70's Show*

Lois from *Malcolm in the Middle*

Morticia Addams from *The Addams Family*

baby before returning to work. Some are going to wonder why a mom decided to return to work at all, while others will ask if a job that pays in precious moments is enough. New moms feel praised and criticized multiple times a day, and sometimes your worst critic will be the tired eyes staring back at you in the mirror (if you're lucky, a fleeting glance at your reflection in the side of a toaster is probably more realistic). Most everyone will realize that being a mom is a lot of work, so take it easy on yourself when you can.

"Trust your inner voice. There are many voices trying to influence your choices as a new mom. There are always fads that come in and out of style. You have to make the best decisions based on your values as a family."

–*Eileen*

GOOD MOTHERS

The important thing to remember is that there is always going to be somebody out there telling us how to be good mothers. It's easy for someone on the outside to offer advice, and sometimes it's helpful, but the relationship we have with our children is private, unique, and special. Think about what being a good mother means to you. What did your own mother do that you'd like to reinstate with your children? What didn't she do that you'd like to do? How can you decipher how to handle the peer pressure? It's important to know that we, by nature, know what to do. We might make mistakes, but as the guidebooks change with the overalls and bell bottoms, our hearts stay clear, certain, and always in style. Love doesn't change, it grows. We love our children, and we love the idea of being new moms.

"When John was first born, I can remember sitting there looking down at him in awe and thinking *wow, we made this human being.* What a wonder, what a beautiful thing. I didn't enjoy being pregnant but it was worth it in the end for sure."

—*Edie*

Pregnancy Journal

I worry that I:

_____

_____

_____

_____

I value my:

_____

_____

_____

_____

It's important that I:

_____

_____

_____

_____

I need to:

_____

_____

_____

_____

_____

I will seek guidance from:

_____

_____

_____

_____

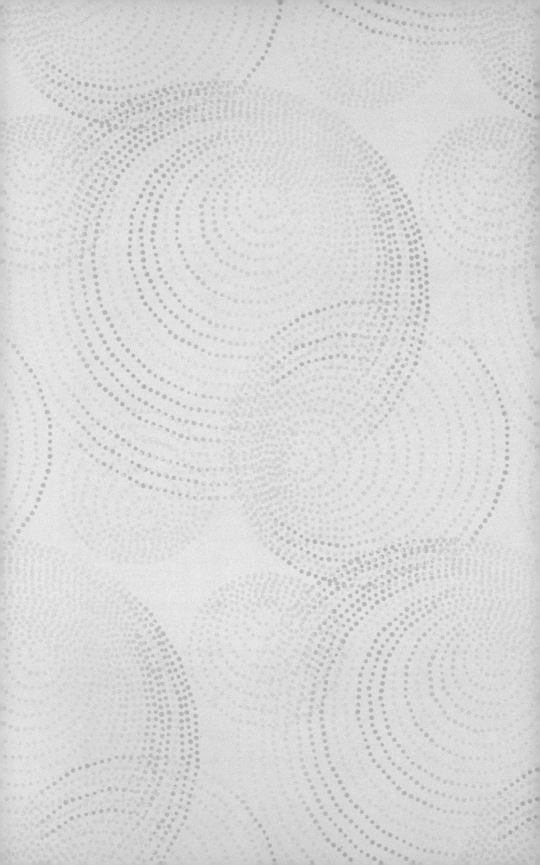

Chapter 8

WHERE BABIES COME FROM

How is it that cartoon storks ended up carrying cute newborn babies from their beaks on greeting cards? Maybe our lives would have been easier if the whole storks-bringing-us-babies thing was true, but we'd have less to complain about, then, and it wouldn't be as special, would it? Kids are going to ask us a lot of questions, and then follow up all of those queries with that one beloved word, "why," one hundred times more. In Victorian England, it's no wonder prude parents resorted to fiction when explaining where babies come from. Storks are friendly to humans and don't scare easily, so they were the perfect storytelling scapegoats.

NEST AND CHILL

If there seems to be a connection between the number of storks in a village and the number of babies born there in any given year, it's because that village probably has a bunch of chimneys for these storks to nest and chill. More chimneys mean more cuddle time by the fireplace. We've all been snowed in before; we know that confinement leads to booze and baby-making. It seems the big sell for the stork as a baby delivery boy began in Germany during warmer months long ago.

SUMMER SOLSTICE STORKS

In Germany, lots of weddings took place during the celebration of the summer solstice. There was plenty of romancing and fertility pumping at the time of Mid-

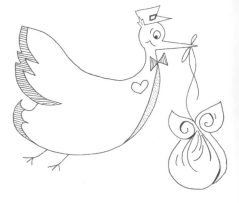

summer's Eve. Pagan holiday marriage celebrations led to baby-making in June, which produced births in March and April the following spring season. At one point, March was considered to be a very lucky time to have a baby! Well, wouldn't you know it? The storks were on a nine-month tour, too. That's precisely when storks returned to Europe from their migratory trek to Africa. They might not have had human babies in tow, but they were giving birth to their own little chicks, becoming symbols of new life.

THE TALE OF THE STORK

The stork has a place in many mythologies, and Hans Christian Anderson did his part to make these big birds notorious in his short story written about them in the nineteenth century. In his tale, angelic storks snagged happily sleeping babies from ponds and estuaries everywhere and delivered them to deserving families. In sparkling, magical ponds, baby souls were just waiting to be collected and handed over to parents yearning for children. Families of well-behaved children would be gifted with a healthy baby, while families with badly-behaved kids were brought something else. We don't have to talk about the punishment part of the story because nobody's kids have perfect behavior and this book is all about love. Sappy, maybe, but nothing sad. Speaking of, here's something sweet! In some countries, people would leave sweets in the window to let the storks know the family was ready to conceive a baby. How cute is that?

Top 10 Nursery Must-Haves

Crib

Bedding for crib

Night light

Comfy chair, Rocking chair, or glider

Dresser with changing table

Baby monitor

Cradle or bassinet

Diaper pail

Mobile

Humidifier

THE NAME GAME

First, we were tasked with creating a child. That was the fun part. Then, we were challenged with carrying that child, and that was the Supermom training. Now, we are employed with naming our child, deciding what to call this beautiful little human and imagining how this epic title will guide them throughout their entire life. With this important job, we must be thoughtful, 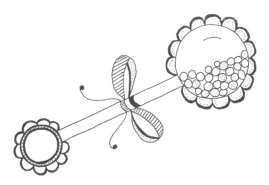 strategic, and realistic. We have a duty, this is our first chance to imagine and tangibly introduce this adorable little creation to the rest of the world.

NAMING RULES AROUND THE WORLD

There is no right or wrong answer when choosing a name, except there might be rules depending on where you live. Not every parent has the luxury of choosing just any quirky name like a Hollywood star. Some countries have laws in place that restrict parents from naming their kids anything that might be deemed bizarre or inappropriate.

AN APPROVED LIST

In Denmark, the spelling of names must follow what is customary and parents can choose from a list of pre-approved names. If you want to name your child something that isn't on the list, you have to get special permission from a local church. Names must be indicative of gender, which is also the case in Iceland. In Iceland and Hungary, parents can choose from a list of baby names.

ICE, ICE, BABY

The National Registry of Persons in Iceland, formed in 1991, decides if a new name will even be acceptable. It must fit grammatically with the language and shouldn't embarrass the poor child once they're old enough to realize their name is undesirable. You also have to apply for approval and pay a fee, just like in Germany.

RESTRICTIONS

Saudi Arabia has a list of banned names based on religious or social traditions. In Europe, you can't name a baby Hitler or Stalin. Japan rejects names that might be inappropriate, and China requires that a child be named based on the ability of computer scanners to read those names on identification cards. New Zealand's Births, Deaths, and Marriages Registration Act of 1995 restricts parents from naming their babies anything unsuitable according to the standards provided. Names can't be too long or offensive.

TIME SENSITIVE

In Australia, you have to give your baby a name within six months of their birth date. The naming law of Sweden prevents non-noble families from giving their children noble names. Pretending to be important will have to be a dress-up game your child plays when they're old enough, but it won't be on their birth certificate.

TRADITIONS

In Bali, there are select names chosen for your first, second, third, and fourth-born children. In Ireland and England, names are provided in a specific birth order according to your family history. Every culture has its own traditions for how to name a baby, and in the United States, each state has its own particular rules and expectations.

NAMING IN THE UNITED STATES

If you're thinking about naming your baby a number, you won't be able to do so in Alabama. You will be able to name your child something that has an apostrophe or hyphen, though. In California, you can't name your child an emoji, and pictographs like smiley faces or symbols like a thumbs-up sign are specifically banned. Does that mean someone actually tried this? Only in Hollywood!

NOBODY PUTS BABY IN A CORNER

In Arkansas, you can have apostrophes, hyphens, or spaces in a name but they can't be consecutive. You'll have to have your baby in another state if you'd like to officially name your child Baby. Some states like Alaska and Arizona can handle foreign characters like tildes, but other locations restrict non-letters. If you have a traditional name in mind you should be A-OK, but if you're thinking outside the box, you might want to check the rules specific to the state where you are giving birth. You don't want to be disappointed when you realize the asterisk you had planned isn't going to work out for Ad*m.

Baby Name Brainstorming

When considering baby names, think about names that have a special meaning to you. Are there any family names you might want to incorporate? Are there real people or fictional characters that have inspired you in some way? Do you prefer any specific letter of the alphabet? Practice writing potential baby names here, and say them out loud a few times too. When you find joy in spelling and saying a particular name, that one might be the keeper!

NAMING ADVICE

Speaking of thinking outside the box, there are definitely realistic things to consider when choosing a name for your baby. We all love the idea of our baby's name being original, unique, and memorable. But think about the reality of your baby living with their given name. Is the name easy to remember? Is it easy to spell and pronounce? Do you really want to have your child tortured every year in school because the teacher can't correctly read your child's name out loud? Before deciding on a name and sticking to it, write out your baby's initials. Do the initials form a word? Are the kids on the school bus able to create an unwanted rhyme or acronym? It's also important to keep in mind that no matter how much you love the name Jonathon, chances are, the world is going to know your son by John. If you don't like the shortened version of a name you adore, you might want to consider choosing something else.

SHORT AND SWEET

It's only natural for people to give other people nicknames. Does the name you have in mind fare well in that regard? On the contrary, does the baby's name remind you of anything weird? Does it remind others of something that is unlikable or unsuitable? Does the name fit a baby and a fully grown adult? Is it cute enough for a little girl and sophisticated enough for a working woman? With so many things to consider, don't lose sleep over it, but think deeply about whether or not you can live with your choice for the long haul.

POPULAR BABY GIRL NAMES

For nearly forty years straight, Mary was the most popular name for a girl in America, from 1918–1946. Mary took second place to Linda from 1946 until 1952, then regained her throne until 1961, when she took second place to Lisa until 1970. The 1970s saw the end of an era with Mary becoming old news and Jennifer stepping in to be Ms. Popular. From 1970 until 1984, Jennifer was the most common baby name for a little girl, only to be outdone by Jessica from 1985 until 1990. Jessica and Ashley split the popularity contest until 1995. That's when Emily rocked it until 2008, with Emma, Isabella, and Sophia taking turns from then on being the most popular names for girls until 2017.

Other female favorites that hit the top five rankings for baby girl names in the past one hundred years were Abigail, Alexis, Amanda, Amy, Angela, Ava, Barbara, Betty, Brittany, Carol, Deborah, Debra, Donna, Dorothy, Hannah, Heather, Helen, Joan, Judith, Karen, Kimberly, Linda, Lisa, Madison, Margaret, Melissa, Michelle, Olivia, Patricia, Ruth, Samantha, Sandra, Sarah, Shirley, and Susan. In a century's time, Mary was ranked in first place thirty-eight times while Michael was the most popular name for a boy forty-four times.

POPULAR BABY BOY NAMES

John was the most popular name for a baby boy from 1918–1923. Then, Robert took over the throne from 1924–1939, when James stepped in from 1940–1952. Robert had a return tour in 1953, but in 1954, Michael began his long reign as the most popular name for a baby boy until 1998. There was one rogue year in 1960 when Michael took second place to David. From 1999 to 2012, baby boys were named Jacob the most, while Noah took first place from 2012 to 2016, and Liam ranked first in 2017. Other well-liked boy names in the past century include Alexander, Andrew, Charles, Christopher, Daniel, Ethan, Jason, Jayden, Joshua, Logan, Mason, Matthew, Richard, Tyler, and William.

Pregnancy Journal

I love the name:

_____
_____
_____
_____
_____

This name was chosen because:

_____
_____
_____
_____
_____

I hope this name:

_____
_____
_____
_____
_____

My baby's nickname will be:

_____

_____

_____

_____

_____

Deciding on a name was:

_____

_____

_____

_____

_____

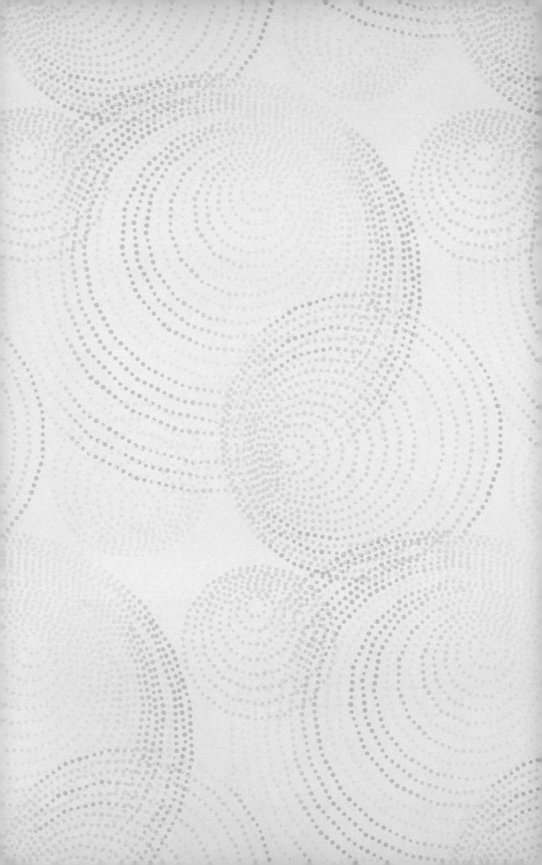

Chapter 9

LABOR OF LOVE

Thank goodness for all of those smart people who wear scrubs, the heaven on Earth angels who have studied childbirth while contemplating and analyzing the sheer mystery of fitting a watermelon through a tiny little hamster-house hose (and surviving without even reflex vomiting). The weather report for our future suggests sunny with the good chance of one meatball emerging from our hoo-ha's! Now that we have settled into the reality that there has been a little human growing inside the cavernous region of our uterine walls, it's time for this baby train to unload and for hot mama to get her groove back.

LABOR INDUCERS

Are there labor inducers that actually work? Apparently, taking a walk doesn't actually induce labor because gravity isn't going to pull the baby out of your vagina. Thank goodness. Could you imagine if gravity worked that way? We'd all be walking around with our hand cupped over our privates. There isn't much evidence or reasoning to support the other ideas of eating pizza, taking a bath, drinking herbal tea, exercising, being scared, or drinking castor oil (yuck). Eating pizza while taking a bath couldn't really hurt though, right? Actually, it turns out there is some scientific evidence to support sex as a labor inducer. It may induce contractions because of a substance found in sperm. Need anyone say more?

PREPARING FOR LABOR

Women describe labor in different ways. It can feel like getting punched in the gut or stabbed in the side, but many say it's not that bad. So, who should we be-

> "I went into the childbirth process without a plan and with an open mind. I tried to get an epidural, but I was too late. Now, I feel like a superhero! Labor is indescribable, but ultimately our bodies were made for it."
>
> —*Caitlin*

lieve? The fact is your own experience is going to be unique to your body, and you are going to make it out just fine. It's like menstrual cramps, but worse? Cool beans. We've all been dealing with cramps for years. We've been constipated, nauseous, and mentally preparing for this event since we were born. Our hips have hurt, no big deal. We've all powered through a night on the town in high heels that don't fit our fat feet. Easy as pie. We've got this.

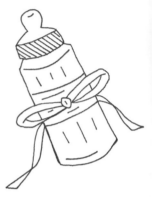

> "I got an epidural with my first. Baby #2 came so fast I didn't have time for an epidural, and I found the recovery time much faster and better; so I chose a natural delivery with baby #3 as well."
>
> —*Jenny*

We can do this! It's not even going to be the hardest thing we'll have to do. It can't be as hard as picking out colors for the nursery or deciding how much to pack for vacation or what to eat for dinner. Nobody is having what we're having today. We're delivering a baby, and nobody can stop us from screaming yelps of . . . joy.

WHAT TO PACK

Now that you have the end of this journey on your mind, you have to prepare. You can do so by thinking about what you'd like to pack in your bag for the hospital. Your partner should also pack a bag because they should be comfortable too. Some items you both might like to include are:

- Something to read like magazines or a Kindle
- A change of clothes (preferably something warm, soft, and snuggly)
- Socks and/or slippers
- A bathrobe or nightgown
- Phones and phone chargers
- Snacks
- Important stuff like a photo ID, insurance information, paperwork

Keep this simple and realistic. You shouldn't go through the same anxiety you experience while packing for an island trip because you don't have to choose between thirty of your cute bikinis.

Top 10 Labor Pain Songs

"Help!" by The Beatles

"The Waiting" by Tom Petty and the Heartbreakers

"Under Pressure" by David Bowie/Queen

"Hold On" by Alabama Shakes

"Hurts So Good" by John Mellencamp

"Good Vibrations" by Marky Mark and the Funky Bunch

"Ring of Fire" by Johnny Cash

"Piece of My Heart" by Janis Joplin

"If I Could Turn Back Time" by Cher

"Love Hurts" by Nazareth

WHAT TO KNOW

While packing, think about including a notebook (or borrow a page from this book). Write down important information about your blood type and Rh factor, when your last period was, your baby's due date, and your doctor's name. Are you sometimes forgetful? Take a picture of that page with your phone! You should also familiarize

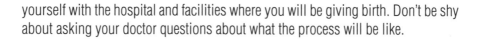

yourself with the hospital and facilities where you will be giving birth. Don't be shy about asking your doctor questions about what the process will be like.

WHAT TO DECIDE

Think about specifics ahead of time. Here are some questions to consider:

- Does your insurance cover the doctor at the hospital?
- What hospital will you be delivering your baby at?
- Is the hospital close to your house?
- Who will be present in the delivery room?
- Do you plan to get an epidural or will you attempt a totally natural child birth?

Epidural anesthesia is a local anesthesia that makes pain in a particular area of the body disappear. Sounds magical, right? It's important to discuss different pain relief options with your doctor ahead of time. Educate yourself on what you think will be the best choice for you before you are at the hospital. You can always change your mind, but it's good practice to have a loose birth plan based on what you know. It's also important to be willing to adapt to make the best choice when you are actually experiencing labor.

"You don't know what your labor will be like so I just suggest keeping an open mind. If you go in thinking you want to do it without an epidural, don't be upset if you decide you need one. Any way you go through labor, it's hard and each woman is amazing and strong for doing it."

–*Kate*

ARRIVAL OF SUPER BABY

Remember how your Supermom training had three stages? Three seems to be the lucky number because labor comes in three stages too (although some say there is a fourth stage). The first part of this whole pushing-a-human-out-of-you adventure begins with uterine contractions. Like any good Tom Cruise action film, these contractions build up intensity, duration, and frequency as we get deeper into labor. They might start out by lasting a minute and not looping back for about twenty minutes. This stage will end with the contractions being stronger and more frequent, coming back every three minutes. It's as if your labor first presents itself as an innocent crush and then later transforms into a Lifetime movie about a stalker that won't leave you alone.

What's more, this stage of labor can last up to twenty hours. Yikes! Don't think about the longevity, think about the light at the end of the birth canal. Take comfort in the fact that stage one is the longest part, so once you get through that, you only have to worry about pushing a giant human head through your tiny elastic vagina. No biggie.

> "You can plan and try to prepare all you can, but when the time comes, all of those plans might be thrown out the window, and that's okay. You just need to not panic and roll with it."
>
> —*Anastasia*

Stage two begins when the cervix is completely dilated at ten centimeters and ends with the delivery of the baby. This part will be a cinch. Just squeeze out the baby like it's no big deal. Stage three begins with the delivery of the baby and ends with the delivery of the cute placenta and all of those adorable membranes that surrounded the fetus and kept it safe all of that time in your belly. In Bali, some Hindus consider the placenta to be alive, like a twin sibling of the newborn baby. As a result, they believe in burying the placenta just to be safe.

After these three pieces of labor pie, some say there is a fourth stage. After the delivery of the baby and placenta, the uterus contracts to control the bleeding that can happen from all of the stuff your body just went through. Once that's done, you just have to figure out how to be a parent. No big deal though—we've got this!

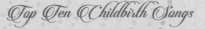

Top Ten Childbirth Songs

"Push It" by Salt N' Pepa

"With Arms Wide Open" by Creed

"Love is a Battlefield" by Pat Benatar

"Let It Go" by Idina Menzel

"Let My Love Open the Door" by Pete Townshend

"SOB" by Nathanial Rateliff and the Night Sweats

"My Baby Left Me" by Elvis

"I Would Do Anything for Love" by Meatloaf

"Free Fallin'" by Tom Petty and the Heartbreakers

"I was Born This Way" by Lady Gaga

A BEAUTIFUL LIFE

The end of your pregnancy means the beginning of a beautiful life. This is when your planning and new mom training starts to kick in. While it's been good to prepare, it's important to realize that some of the most important parenting moments cannot be practiced. Baby is going to poop when baby wants to poop. Baby will sleep when baby feels like it. We might be the teachers meant to guide our little ones, but sometimes, our babies may become the best tutors as we grow into motherhood. Each day you get through with your baby is a victory. Don't sweat the small stuff and embrace all of the moments—even the icky ones. Let the giggles energize you, the little feet lead you, and the gross snots keep you humble.

"All I want to do is keep them safe and make sure that they're happy, and I can't be happy unless I know that they are. The way they look at me when I do something as simple as open a toy wrapper or reach a cup from the top shelf for them makes me feel like I'm doing something real in my life."

—*Anastasia*

BRINGING BABY HOME

There's been a lot of pep talk about becoming Supermom, and all of it is true. There's also truth to the fact that you probably aren't going to feel like Supermom for quite some time. You might feel drained. You might feel down. Heck, you're bound to be exhausted, confused, and terrified. In other moments, you might be elated. You might feel like you are flying on cloud nine. No matter what, you will be in love, and we all know that love is not an easy thing. It challenges us in ways we could never imagine, but the ascension is what makes it magnificent. The fall is what helps us grow. The unexplainable, downright flooring sensation in the pit of our stomachs grounds us into better people. The little light that fuels our hearts, lifts our spirits, and cues the tears in our eyes is a warm guide we so desperately need. The twinkle gives us wings! Whatever you are feeling, at any given moment, take a deep breath and let love guide you. Congratulations, my dearest mommy-to-be! You've joined the ranks of many strong women that came before you, and your time to be is now. Breathe in each moment. You are going to be amazing. You are going to be you—and you have the makings to be the best kind of mom.

"This feeling is kind of indescribable for me. It's like you wait the nine months for your baby to be born. You go through the whole process of delivering the baby, having contractions, pain, etc., and then you hear your baby's cry and any pain or discomfort you may have experienced becomes a fond memory."

—Judy

Pregnancy Journal

Labor was:

_____

_____

_____

_____

My doctor was:

_____

_____

_____

_____

I always want to remember:

_____

_____

_____

_____

I'd kind of like to forget:

_____

_____

_____

_____

I'm so in love with:

_____

_____

_____

_____

Dream Team Stats

Date of birth:

_____

_____

_____

_____

Time of birth:

_____

_____

_____

_____

Baby's weight:

_____

_____

_____

_____

Baby's length:

_____

_____

_____

_____

_____

Time in labor:

_____

_____

_____

_____

_____

Baby's Hand and Feet Prints

Baby's Hand and Feet Prints

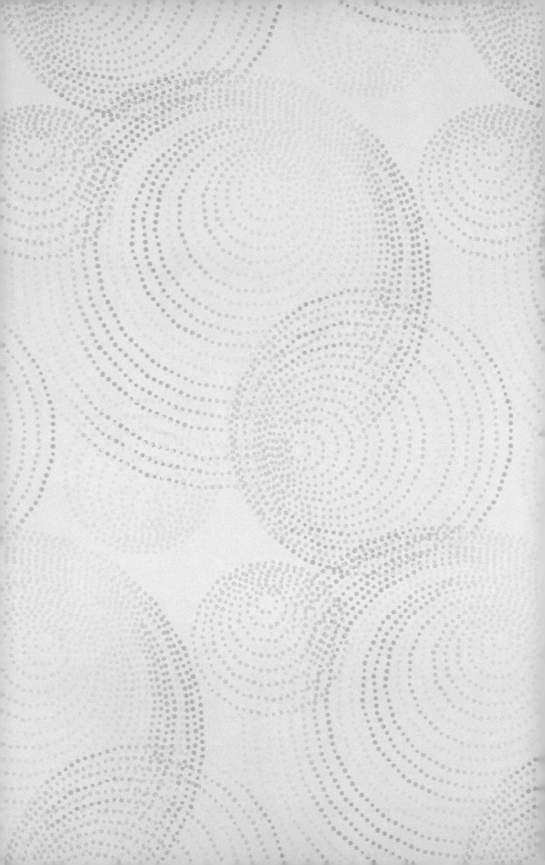

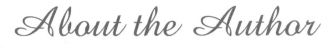

About the Author

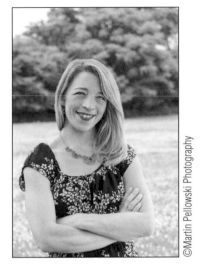

©Martin Pellowski Photography

Melanie J. Pellowski is a happily married journalist, author, and educator who looks forward to one day starting a family with her husband, Nick. She has always considered motherhood to be one of the most important, valuable, and challenging jobs for women, especially in today's busy world. The special bond she has with her own mother, Judy, began before she was born, continues today, and served as the inspiration for this book.

A family mindset has always been at the core of Melanie's developing career. Her three brothers, Morgan, Matthew, and Martin, have each played a significant role in her life both creatively and professionally. Her father, Michael, is an accomplished author who has often provided valued mentorship on many of Melanie's writing projects.

Melanie graduated Phi Beta Kappa from Douglass College, Rutgers University in 2005 with a major in American Studies and minors in Mathematics and Theatre Arts. She earned a master's degree in journalism from Boston University in 2008. Throughout many stages in her life, including high school athletics and her sorority days at Rutgers, Melanie feels lucky to have developed friendships and professional relationships with unique, well-rounded women. She has seen many of her dearest friends and family members embrace the role of becoming new moms, and she has written *Pregnancy Primer* with all of these strong female role models in mind.

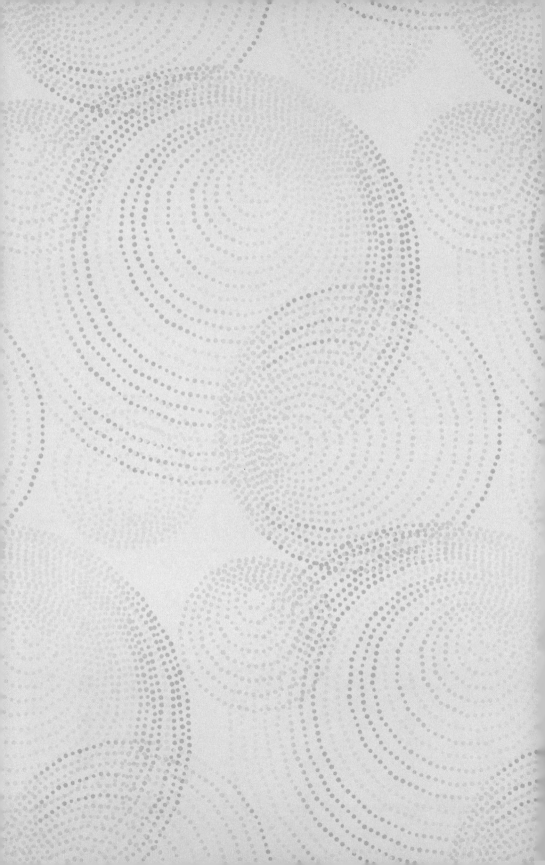

Acknowledgments

This book was inspired by a strong and diverse group of women who share a bond in motherhood but are distinguished by their own personal take on such an important role. Having not yet had the opportunity to become a mom myself at the time of writing this book, I relied heavily on dear friends, family members, and colleagues who I greatly respect and admire. Being able to see the process of pregnancy and motherhood through their eyes not only helped me craft a deeper understanding of the bond between a mommy and her children, but it eased my own personal anxieties about what becoming a mom will mean in my own life. Their advice and individual perspectives made me even more excited to start a family. Thank you to all of the moms who took time away from their busy lives to respond to my questions. Anastasia, Caitlin, Casey, Christy, Edie, Gabby, Kate, Jackie, and Jenny: You not only provided helpful tips on being great caregivers, but you are equally influential in your careers, crafts, cooking skills, and character. Thank you to my mother-in-law, Eileen, for always being so supportive and insightful. Thank you to my mom, Judy, for your love, guidance, and friendship. I continue to be inspired by all of the shopping trips, crafting tips, and mother-daughter adventures. My heart is full. This may be a mom book, but I have to also thank my father, Michael, and my husband, Nick, who both spent countless hours discussing ideas and providing creative consultations. Finally, thank you to Nicole Mele and Skyhorse Publishing for making the publication of *Pregnancy Primer* possible.

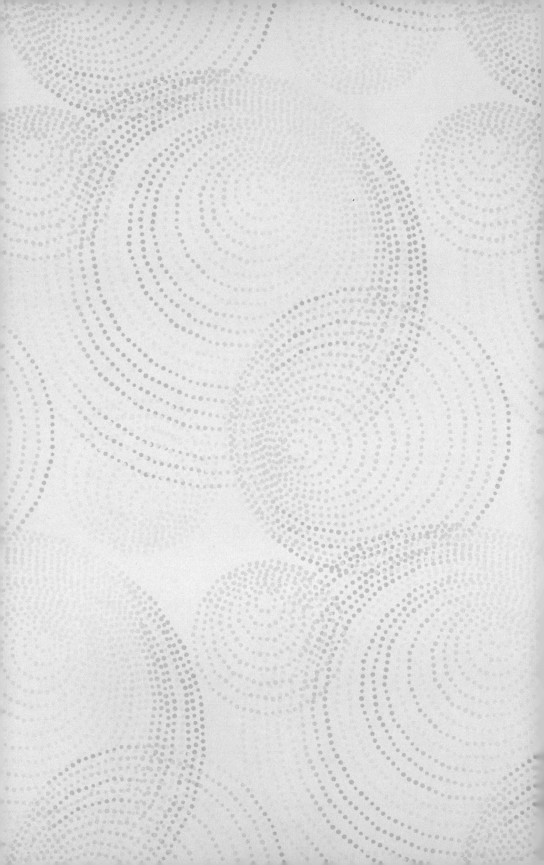

Bibliography

"11 Unique Birthing Traditions Around the World." *Huffington Post.* 6 Dec. 2017, huffpost.com/entry/world-birthing-traditions_n_7033790. Accessed Dec. 2018.

Ahmed, Sarah. "49 Great Moms in History Who More than Left their Mark." *Babble.* babble.com/entertainment/famous-moms-in-history. Accessed Dec. 2018.

Ambar, Saladin. "Woodrow Wilson: Life Before the Presidency." *Miller Center.* millercenter.org/president/wilson/life-before-the-presidency. Accessed Jan. 2019.

"Births, Deaths, Marriages, and Relationships Registration Act 1995." *New Zealand Registration.* legislation.govt.nz/act/public/1995/0016/73.0/DLM364129.html. Accessed Dec. 2018.

"Baby Shower Beginnings: How it All Started." *Babies Online.* babiesonline.com /articles/pregnancy/baby-showers/baby-shower-beginnings.asp. Accessed Jan. 2019.

Bryce, Emma. "What's Behind the Myth that Storks Deliver Babies?" *Live Science.* 13 Jun. 2018, livescience.com/62807-why-storks-baby-myth.html. Accessed Jan. 2019.

Brody, Susan. "Pregnancy Cravings." *Parents.* parents.com/pregnancy/my-body/ nutrition/pregnancy-cravings. Accessed Jan. 2019.

Coleman, Patrick A. "How Babies Are Traditionally Named in 8 Countries, from India to Iceland." *Fatherly.* 16 Aug. 2016, fatherly.com/health-science/baby-naming-traditions -around-world. Accessed Dec. 2018.

Curtis, Glade B., M.D., OB/GYN and Judith Schuler, M.S. *Your Pregnancy Week by Week: Fourth Edition.* Cambridge, MA: Fisher Books, 2000.

Cieslik, Anna. "Cabinet of Curiosities: What Really Causes Pregnancy Cravings?" *Daily Break.* 7 Nov. 2017, dailybreak.com/break/why-do-pregnant-women-get -intense-cravings. Accessed Jan. 2019.

Cieslik, Anna. "Cabinet of Curiosities: Why We Tell Kids that the Stork Brought their Baby Sibling." *Daily Break.* 10 Jan. 2018, dailybreak.com/break/where-does -the-myth-of-storks-delivering-babies-come-from. Accessed Jan. 2019.

Coontz, Stephanie. "When We Hated Mom." *The New York Times.* 7 May 2011, nytimes.com/2011/05/08/opinion/08coontz.html. Accessed Jan. 2019.

Cronin, Melissa. "7 Astonishing Animal Moms Who Prove Mother's Day Shouldn't Be Reserved for People." *The Dodo.* 9 May 2014, thedodo.com/7-astonishing -animal-moms-who—543168457.html. Accessed Dec. 2018.

Debczak, Michele. "22 Outlawed Baby Names from Around the World." *Mental Floss.* 28 Mar. 2017, mentalfloss.com/article/68768/22-outlawed-baby-names -around-world. Accessed Jan. 2019.

Dove, Laurie L. "You Can't Name Your Baby That!" *How Stuff Works.* 18 May 2018, health.howstuffworks.com/pregnancy-and-parenting/you-cant-name-your -baby-that.htm. Accessed Dec. 2018.

"Do Storks Deliver Babies?" *Priceonomics.* priceonomics.com/do-storks-deliver -babies. Accessed Jan. 2019.

Deasey, Louisa. "Funny but True: Old Wives' Tales About Pregnancy." *Kid Spot.* 3 Feb. 2012, kidspot.com.au/birth/pregnancy/pregnancy-health/funny-but-true-old -wives-tales-about-pregnancy/news-story/7f6048a0813bd6e8363f40515f-1c3a36. Accessed Jan. 2019.

Drewes, Lindsay. "14 Old Wives' Tales About Pregnancy that are Actually True." *Baby Gaga.* 28 Jan. 2017, babygaga.com/14-old-wives-tales-about-pregnancy -that-are-actually-true. Accessed Jan. 2018.

Elliot, Kristine. "A Brief Introduction to the History of Names." *SCA College of Arms.* 1997, heraldry.sca.org/names/namehist.html. Accessed Dec. 2018.

Evans, Cleveland Kent. "Baby Naming Trends." *How Stuff Works.* lifestyle.how-stuffworks.com/family/parenting/babies/baby-name-trends-ga.htm. Accessed Dec. 2018.

Erbland, Kate. "11 Awesome Animal Kingdom Moms." *Mental Floss.* 9 May 2014, mentalfloss.com/article/56604/11-awesome-animal-kingdom-moms. Accessed Jan. 2019.

Faber, Doris. *The Mothers of American Presidents.* New York, New York: The New American Library, Inc., 1968.

"Food Cravings and What They Mean." *Baby Center.* May 2016. babycenter. com/0_food-cravings-and-what-they-mean_1313971.bc. Accessed Jan. 2019.

Gammon, Katherine. "The 7 Weirdest Moms in the Animal Kingdom." *Live Science*. 11 May 2014, livescience.com/45496-weirdest-animal-moms.html. Accessed Jan. 2019.

Gibbons, Layne A. "20 Old Wives Tales Our Mothers Were Told About Birth." *Moms*. 26 Jul. 2018, moms.com/20-old-wives-tales-our-mothers-were-told-about-birth. Accessed Dec. 2018.

Gilbert, Sarah Emily. "Best Moms in the Animal Kingdom." *Princeton Magazine*. princetonmagazine.com/best-moms-in-the-animal-kingdom. Accessed Jan. 2019.

Granger, Sarah. "14 Questions to Ask Your Care Provider." *Pregnancy & Newborn*. pnmag.com/pregnancy/prenatal-care/14-questions-to-ask-your-care-provider-2. Accessed Dec. 2018.

Handwerk, Brian. "7 Things You Don't Know About Mother's Day's Dark History." *National Geographic*. 10 May 2017, news.nationalgeographic.com/2015/05/150507 -mothers-day-history-holidays-anna-jarvis. Accessed Jan. 2019.

Hartmann, Margaret. "The History of Pink for Girls, Blue for Boys." *Jezebel*. 10 Apr. 2011, jezebel.com/the-history-of-pink-for-girls-blue-for-boys-5790638. Accessed Dec. 2018.

"The History of the Baby Shower." *Little Things & Favors*. littlethingsfavors.com/baby -shower-history.html. Accessed Jan. 2019.

Hutson, Stacey. "How the Role of Being a Mom Has Changed Throughout History." *The List*. thelist.com/58638/how-role-mom-changed-throughout-history. Accessed Jan. 2019.

Israel, David K. "8 Countries with Fascinating Baby Naming Laws." *Mental Floss*. 28 June 2010, mentalfloss.com/article/25034/8-countries-fascinating-baby-naming -laws. Accessed Dec. 2018.

Koutsky, Judy. "Checkmate." *Pregnancy & Newborn*. pnmag.com/pregnancy/prenatal -care/checkmate-2. Accessed Dec. 2018.

Lambert, Laura. "Blame the Book: Parenting by Decade." *Brightly*. readbrightly.com /blame-book-parenting-decade. Accessed Dec. 2018.

Langley, Liz. "6 Fierce Animal Moms that Go to Extremes for their Young." *National Geographic*. 13 May 2017, news.nationalgeographic.com/2017/05/animals-mothers -pandas-spiders-octopus. Accessed Jan. 2019.

Maglaty, Jeanne. "When Did Girls Start Wearing Pink?" *Smithsonian.* 7 Apr. 2011, smithsonianmag.com/arts-culture/when-did-girls-start-wearing-pink-1370097. Accessed Dec. 2018.

Matthews, Robert. "Storks Deliver Babies (p = 0.008)." *Aston University.* Summer 2000, robertmatthews.org/wp-content/uploads/2016/03/RM-storks-paper.pdf. Accessed Dec. 2018.

Mauer, Elena Donovan. "5 Ways Pets Can Be Bad (or Good!) for You and Baby." *The Bump.* thebump.com/a/pets-pregnancy. Accessed Jan. 2019.

Miles, Tiya. "Baby Showers, Now and Then." *Huffington Post.* 25 Aug. 2014, huffpost.com/entry/baby-showers-now-and-then_b_5527222. Accessed Jan. 2019.

Mintz, Steven. "Decade by Decade: Snapshots of Motherhood from 1890—Present. *The Mother Company.* 6 May 2015, themotherco.com/2015/05/decade-by-decade-a-snapshot-of-motherhood-from-1890-present. Accessed Dec. 2018.

"The Most Amazing Moms in the Animal Kingdom." *Ripley's Believe It or Not.* 8 May 2018, ripleys.com/weird-news/animal-moms. Accessed Dec. 2018.

Murkoff, Heidi and Sharon Mazel. *What to Expect When You're Expecting: Fourth Edition.* New York, New York: Workman Publishing, 2008.

"Naming Children: Traditions in 13 Different Countries." *Pocket Cultures.* 13 Apr. 2011, pocketcultures.com/2011/04/13/children-naming-traditions. Accessed Dec. 2018.

"Naming Traditions and Ceremonies from Around the World." *Confetti: Celebrate in Style.* 12 Mar. 2007, confetti.co.uk/wedding-advice/relationships/naming-traditions-and-ceremonies-from-around-the-world. Accessed Dec. 2018.

Norris, Anna. "15 of the Hardest-Working Moms in the Animal Kingdom." *MNN.* 7 May 2014, mnn.com/earth-matters/animals/stories/15-of-the-hardest-working-moms-in-the-animal-kingdom. Accessed Jan. 2019.

"Old Wives' Tales Baby's Gender." *Huggies.* huggies.com.au/pregnancy/early-stages/gender-prediction/old-wives-tales. Accessed Jan. 2019.

"The Origin of the Baby Shower." *My Baby Bakery.* mybabybakery.com/blog/77. Accessed Jan. 2018.

Pappas, Stephanie. "5 Ways Motherhood Has Changed Over Time." *Live Science*. 10 May 2013, livescience.com/29521-5-ways-motherhood-has-changed.html. Accessed Dec. 2018.

Pappas, Stephanie. "Why Pregnancy Really Lasts Nine Months." *Live Science*. 27 Aug. 2012, livescience.com/22715-pregnancy-length-baby-size.html. Accessed Jan. 2019.

Pianegonda, Elise. "If a Baby Isn't Named within a Certain Period of Time, Can the ACT Government Name a Child?" *ABC*. 20 Sept. 2017, abc.net.au/news/specials /curious-canberra/2017-09-18/can-the-act-government-name-a-child/8949402. Accessed Dec. 2018.

"Popular Baby Names." *Social Security*. https://www.ssa.gov/oact/babynames/. Accessed 5 Jan. 2019.

"Pregnancy Advice: Old Wives' Tales vs. Science." *Parents*. parents.com/pregnancy /my-body/pregnancy-health/pregnancy-advice-old-wives-vs-science. Accessed Jan. 2019.

"Pregnancy and Pica." *American Pregnancy Association*. americanpregnancy.org /pregnancy-health/unusual-cravings-pica. Accessed Jan. 2019.

Przecha, Donna. "The Importance of Names and Naming Patterns: Why are Names Important and What Can You Learn from a First Name?" *Genealogy*. genealogy .com/articles/research/35_donna.html. Accessed Dec. 2018.

Raga, Suzanne. "25 of History's Greatest Moms." *Mental Floss*. 8 May 2016, mentalfloss .com/article/79143/25-historys-greatest-moms. Accessed Dec. 2018.

Ramnarace, Cynthia. "Craziest Baby Naming Laws by State." *The Bump*. thebump .com/a/baby-name-rules. Accessed Dec. 2018.

Sadler, Emily. "12 Old Wives' Tales for Predicting Gender." *Today's Parent*. 25 Jan. 2017, todaysparent.com/pregnancy/9-old-wives-tales-for-predicting-gender. Accessed Dec. 2018.

Sanfilippo, Elizabeth. "10 Best Pregnancy Old Wives' Tales." *Care*. 12 Sept. 2013, care.com/c/stories/4929/10-best-pregnancy-old-wives-tales. Accessed Dec. 2018.

Schalken, Lara. "Birth Customs Around the World." *Parents*. parents.com/pregnancy /giving-birth/vaginal/birth-customs-around-the-world. Accessed Dec. 2018.

Scherer, Jule. "Terrible Parenting Advice from the 1920's." *Stuff.* 10 Oct. 2016, stuff.co.nz/life-style/parenting/baby/caring-for-baby/85019454/terrible-parenting -advice-from-the-1920s. Accessed Jan. 2019.

"She's Something Fierce: Our Favorite Moms of the Animal Kingdom." *Uncommon Goods.* 9 May 2018, uncommongoods.com/blog/2018/coolest-moms-of -the-animal-kingdom. Accessed Jan. 2019.

Smallwood, Jillian. "The First Trimester Blues." *Pregnancy & Newborn.* pnmag .com/pregnancy/prenatal-care/the-first-trimester-blues. Accessed Dec. 2018.

Spears, Nina. "20 Old Wives' Tales to Predict a Baby's Gender." *Baby Chick.* 3 Jan. 2019, baby-chick.com/old-wives-tales-babys-gender. Accessed Jan. 2019.

"Study Up: Pregnancy Vocab You Need to Know." *Pregnancy Magazine.* pregnan-cymagazine.com/pregnancy/pregnancy-vocab-words. Accessed Dec. 2018.

"Top Five Names in Each of the Last 100 Years." *Social Security.* ssa.gov/oact /babynames/top5names.html. Accessed Jan. 2019.

Washney, Rebecca. "5 Ways to Ease the Quease." *Pregnancy & Newborn.* pnmag .com/pregnancy/prenatal-care/5-ways-to-ease-the-quease. Accessed Dec. 2018.

Wasserman, Gary. "The Mama's Boys Who Became Our Presidents." *The Washington Post.* 12 May 1985, washingtonpost.com/archive/opinions/1985/05/12 /the-mamas-boys-who-became-our-presidents/6bf7e1fe-ae53-482d-93eb-7cc802afeeeb/?noredirect=on&utm_term=.3b2cab2efd8b. Accessed Jan. 2019.

"Why Storks Are Associated with Delivering Babies." *Today I Found Out.* 13 May 2013, todayifoundout.com/index.php/2013/05/why-storks-are-associated-with -delivering-babies. Accessed Jan. 2019.

Williams, Geoff. "Debunking Old Wives' Tales About Pregnancy." *Parenting.* parenting .com/article/debunking-pregnancy-old-wives-tales. Accessed Jan. 2019.

Winder, Andy. "15 Scientific Reasons We Monitor Pregnancy the Way We Do." *Baby Gaga.* 25 Feb. 2017, babygaga.com/15-scientific-reasons-we-measure-pregnancy-the-way-we-do. Accessed Dec. 2018.

"Your Pregnancy Checklist: How to Prepare for a Baby." *Parents.* parents.com /pregnancy/my-life/preparing-for-baby/your-pregnancy-checklist. Accessed Dec. 2018.